S0-DGI-477

S. Gibson

*How
Long
Will I
Live?*

HOW LONG WILL I LIVE?

and 434 other questions your doctor doesn't have time to answer and you can't afford to ask

Lawrence Galton

How Long Will I Live? was created by Alan Landsburg Productions, Inc.

Macmillan Publishing Co., Inc.
NEW YORK

Copyright © 1976 by Alan Landsburg Productions Inc.

All rights reserved. No part of this book may be
reproduced or transmitted in any form or by
any means, electronic or mechanical, including
photocopying, recording or by any information
storage and retrieval system, without permission
in writing from the Publisher.

Macmillan Publishing Co., Inc.
866 Third Avenue, New York, N.Y. 10022
Collier Macmillan Canada, Ltd.

Library of Congress Cataloging in Publication
Data

Galton, Lawrence.
    How long will I live?

    Bibliography: p.
    Includes index.
        1. Medicine, Popular.   I. Title.   [DNLM:
1. Health.   2. Medicine—Popular works.
WB130   G181h]
RC82.G33   613   76–2440
ISBN 0–02–542390–8

FIRST PRINTING 1976

Printed in the United States of America

*To
Kit,
Jill,
Jeremy,
their mother
and mine*

Contents

*How
Long
Will I
Live?*

1

Personal Potential

Two propositions lie behind this book. One is that most of us know little about ourselves and what influences how long and how well we'll live. Most people probably know more about their cars than they do about themselves, in terms of the working parts, life expectancy, and how best to care for the machine.

The second proposition is equally simple. Learning about ourselves can be interesting and rewarding and can have elements of fun in it.

Certainly, everything is not yet known about what influences health and longevity, but a surprising amount of information *is* available. The range of influences is broad: from familial predispositions to season and order of birth; from body type to personality type and specific behavior patterns; from sex and sex activity to the place one lives, the work one does, and one's social and marital status.

There are other influences—and, because each of us is different, the combination of influences in our lives is specifically ours.

"You'll go when your number comes up!" is a fatalistic saying common among soldiers. But many other people share this fatalism. To be sure, staying alive and whole may be entirely a matter of chance when war, accident, or natural catastrophe is involved. But for most of us death comes early because of influences not completely beyond our control.

How long should human life be? Nobody really knows. The

oldest living things are trees; perhaps the oldest among them is a bald cypress in Tula, Mexico, believed to be almost 7,000 years old. Animals, in comparison, generally are short-lived. Some tortoises may live to 150 years, but the average life-span is only about fifteen years for dogs, sixteen for bears, twenty-six for chimpanzees and orangutans, thirty for cattle, and seventy-five for elephants.

For most of the one or more million years man has existed, his average life expectancy has not been much more than twenty years. As late as the nineteenth century it was still only about thirty-five; in 1900 it was forty-five; and currently in North America, Europe, Russia, Japan, and a few other places it is about seventy years.

Of all the people who have *ever* reached the age of sixty-five, 25 percent are alive today. As of 1970 there were 11,765,000 people over age seventy in the world. But while more people are living to older age, the life-span has not been extended. Once past forty-five, life expectancy is not much greater than it was in 1900. A man of forty-five can now expect to live to seventy-two, a gain of only three years over 1900; a woman of the same age can expect to live to seventy-seven, a gain of seven years.

Medicine, considerably aided by sanitation as well as wonder drugs, has done a good job in combating the infectious diseases that once killed off large numbers at early ages. But in their place we have the chronic diseases that cripple and kill somewhat later. Against these, medicine has made some progress but not nearly enough.

A long and healthy life, as things stand now, is not a matter solely of medicine. Sweden has 83 doctors per 100,000 population as against 140 per 100,000 in the United States. Yet Sweden has half the death rate among middle-aged men, despite the fact that Americans go to their doctors twice as often as Swedes do.

There are, and always have been, those who happen to have, or pick, the right influences for long and healthy living. When he died in 1635, Thomas Parr, a Shropshire farmer, was reputed to be 152. Joseph Burrington, who died in 1790 at Bergen, Norway, was reported to be 160. A woman who died in Knoxville, Tennessee, in 1935 was supposed to be 154. While there has been some skepticism about these cases for lack of adequate documentation, authenticated records have begun to become available in recent years. When, for example, Louise K. Thiers died in 1926 in Milwaukee, there was satisfactory evidence that she had reached the ripe age of 111 years and 138 days.

Of late, medical investigators have become impressed not only with the wide variations between people in length of life but also with the differences in vigor and health at all ages. In heart-function tests, for example, they have been finding some eighty-year-olds who perform as well as the average forty-year-old.

Some sanguine scientists today foresee an eventual extension of the human life-span to 200 and even 300 years as the result of fundamental new discoveries about old age and aging. Dr. C. W. Hall, a surgeon formerly with the DeBakey team in Houston, now head of the artificial-organs program of Southwest Research Institute, San Antonio, Texas, believes the time has come to start worrying about a whole series of problems likely to result from such extension of the life-span. When, for example, should pensions start if people are going to live to be 200 or 300? What's going to happen to life insurance? What should be the relationship between a child and his 200-year-old, great-to-the-sixth-power grandfather?

Such problems and future possibilities aside, many eminent investigators in the field of gerontology—the study of aging—are convinced that within the next twenty-five years, it will be possible to extend human life—and vigorous life at that—by as much as 20 percent through the use of simple, practical methods.

In question-and-answer format, this book presents useful, individually applicable facts about your body and your life-style. Its goal is to help you live to your own advantage.

2

Family
History

To be long-lived, must one be born into a long-lived family?

No, but it helps. Almost everybody has heard of a family in which many members live to advanced age, perhaps surpassing ninety or even one hundred years. Anyone born into such a family has a lot going for him in the way of potentiality for long life.

People with long-lived forebears tend to have lower mortality rates at every age and a greater chance of reaching or passing the fourscore mark. Whatever a person's present age—twenty-five, thirty-five, fifty, or more—his life expectancy is likely to be greatest if both his parents reached eighty. If they died early, say, before sixty-five, his chances are below average. If their ages at death fell in between the extremes, or one parent was long-lived and the other died early, chances for long life are about average.

So it's a good idea to choose long-lived ancestors. But if you didn't, you're not necessarily doomed. For one thing, the circumstances under which your ancestors died—and lived—have to be considered. Allowance has to be made for deaths due to accidental circumstances; they don't count. Moreover, environmental influences have to be taken into account. Families living through generation after generation of poverty or other unfavorable circumstances would not have the same rate of life expectancy—

4

regardless of inherited traits—as others living under more favorable conditions.

Life expectancy for many people in the past was reduced by environmental conditions rather than by genes. This is still true for many peoples living in underdeveloped countries. An American or European has, at birth, an expectation of living to seventy or beyond; a Burmese or Indian, only to about forty.

Of course heredity has considerable influence on health and longevity, but it is not usually the most important influence. There is no gene that controls how long anyone lives. The most impressive pedigree of long-lived ancestors is not a guarantee against a modern plague such as heart disease. Men whose fathers and grandfathers lived into their eighties and nineties may find themselves victims of heart attacks in their mid-fifties. Also, any apparently "familial" proneness—for example, heart disease occurring in brothers and sisters—has to be viewed with some skepticism. It's not uncommon—in fact it's usual—for family members to share eating and sociological patterns, making it difficult to distinguish acquired from inherited factors. It is often said that the longer husbands and wives live together, the more they tend to look alike. This bit of folklore suggests the influence of common environment.

Is it true that husbands and wives grow to look alike?

There's some scientific evidence that couples do tend to resemble each other—internally, that is. University of Alabama investigators recently checked a sizable group of dentists and their spouses for biochemical levels of blood cholesterol, blood proteins, enzymes, and so on. They correlated the findings between spouses and matched them against the findings for spouses of other dentists. Presumably, they argued, similar biochemical levels among married couples would be due to environmental factors. Sure enough, they found high correlations between spouses but not between dentists and other dentists or the two groups of spouses. And with age biochemical levels for husbands and wives came closer together.

The study, say the investigators, provides evidence that "more emphasis should be placed on environmental factors in predictive medicine programs. Although it may be difficult to alter the environment, it is not as difficult as trying to alter the genetic states. . . . This approach also minimizes the element of hopelessness engendered when diseases are ascribed to purely hereditary factors."

What about race? Are there inherently long-lived races and short-lived ones?

No. Whole peoples can't be separated from their customs and environment any more than individuals can.

A few generations ago "inferior" heredity was said to be the reason why blacks had shorter life expectancies than whites. But as black people have advanced economically the difference between their life expectancy and that of whites has been shrinking. In 1900 the average life expectancy of a newborn nonwhite American was only 33.8 years—fully sixteen years less than that of a white American. But by 1967 the nonwhite life expectancy had risen to 64.6 years and was five years less than that of whites. The life expectancy of a black American not only is greater now than what expectancy once was for whites in this country but also it is greater than current life expectancy of whites in some other countries.

Isn't it true that genetic differences exist among the races?

They do. Differences between population groups are not all traceable to environment. For example, heredity accounts to a considerable degree for the extreme difference in stature between the Pygmies in the Congo and the very tall Dinka people in Sudan.

One area in which genetic differences are studied is the new field of pharmacogenetics, which has to do with the relationship between one's hereditary body chemistry and the way one responds to drugs.

One of the earliest pharmacogenetic reactions recognized occurred during the Korean War when some black American soldiers suddenly became anemic after swallowing an antimalarial agent called primaquine. Investigators found that the anemia results from a deficiency of an enzyme called G6PD in the red cells and that 10 percent of American blacks have this deficiency. They become anemic only when they take drugs like primaquine, sulfa compounds, or headache relievers that contain phenacetin.

Both Indians and Eskimos seem to be affected severely by alcohol. Starting in the days of the early explorers, reports describe alcohol's effects on these people. More recently, in Canada, the continuing importance of drinking as a cause of sickness and death among Indians and Eskimos has been noted. Medical and law enforcement reports indicate that when Indians are jailed while drunk, they take much longer to sober up than do whites.

Some University of Alberta investigators checked on the rate of metabolism of alcohol in the different races. By giving groups of subjects measured drinks and then measuring the alcohol concentration in the blood at various intervals, they found that Indians, Eskimos, and whites required about the same amount of alcohol per unit of body weight in order to get drunk, but that blood concentration of alcohol fell much faster in whites. Neither previous experience with alcohol nor diet accounted for the difference, leaving genetic difference as the likely cause.

Are there racial differences in diseases and defects?

Racial differences exist, but they're generally differences in frequency rather than all-or-none differences. For example, the incidence of color blindness is about 8 percent for white Americans and Europeans, but it's less than one-tenth of one percent for Eskimos. Extra fingers are seven times as frequent among black as among white babies, but the occurrence of mongolian idiocy and harelip is much higher among whites.

Such conditions, however, may not be invariably genetic. Environmental conditions within the womb may be responsible. This possibility is demonstrated with particular clarity by research on harelip, which is establishing that this seemingly inherited abnormality may be produced by hormone, nutritional, drug, or other disturbances in the mother's body chemistry during pregnancy.

When it comes to such life-threatening conditions as heart disease, cancer, and diabetes, frequencies do differ among racial and ethnic groups. But whether inherited factors are involved or not, environmental influences are under suspicion. For example, studies among racial groups in Hawaii have shown varying incidences for different types of cancer and also have suggested possible nongenetic influences. In Hawaii breast cancer is five times more frequent among white women than among Japanese women—could it be because of differences in breast-feeding patterns? Japanese men in Hawaii have a far higher incidence of stomach cancer than other men there—is diet the reason? Prostate cancer is nine times more common among white men than among Japanese men; are differences in sex habits the cause? Japanese living in Hawaii and tending to adopt the local diet and customs have a higher incidence of coronary attacks than do Japanese living in the home islands (and Japanese living in the United States have a still higher incidence).

Jewish people are supposed to be particularly prone to heart disease. But the Yemenites in Israel, whose diet and living patterns differ markedly from those of the European Jews there, have about one-third the prevalence of heart disease.

How many diseases and defects are influenced by heredity?

Some 500, Dr. Victor A. McKusick of Johns Hopkins University has estimated. They include muscular dystrophy, some types of epilepsy, several types of mental retardation, cystic fibrosis, several varieties of blindness and deafness, and some metabolic disorders.

While many malformations present at birth including some heart defects, have been attributed to heredity, leading investigators in congenital malformation research now estimate that only 20 percent of defects are primarily due to hereditary factors, 20 percent are due chiefly to environmental influences, and the remaining 60 percent result from combinations of hereditary and environmental factors.

How can heredity play a role in heart disease?

Heredity may contribute two conditions that could to some extent predispose to heart and artery disease. One is the structure of the blood vessels. If smaller vessels are inherited, they may become clogged more readily by deposits on their inner walls (atherosclerosis), which narrow their bore. Also, heredity may influence the body's metabolism of food. Faulty metabolism, leading to a buildup of abnormal levels of fatty materials in the blood, may foster the atherosclerotic process.

According to some studies, a family history of heart attacks appears to double the risk of heart attack. But, for perspective, consider that hypertension (high blood pressure) alone can mean as much as a 6-to-1 increase in risk; obesity, as much as a 3-to-1 greater risk; and heavy cigarette smoking, up to a 6-to-1 greater risk.

And in cancer?

In the more common forms of cancer, the exact role of heredity is difficult to establish. Cancer is not a specific disease; the term includes any abnormal speedup of cell growth and disruption of normal cell mechanisms. As cells become abnormal, they no longer take an orderly part in body processes but multiply, invade, and destroy neighboring cells and tissues and eventually spread throughout the body.

Environmental factors by the hundreds are known to instigate the conversion of normal cells to malignant ones. These factors are irritants, termed carcinogens, that include a wide variety of chemicals, dusts, and radiations. Viruses are strongly suspect; they have been shown to produce cancers in animals. Research suggests that viruses may be present in the body in dormant state, present even at birth, and they may stay harmless until some disturbance jolts them into action.

Some cancers have been linked to heredity—for example, the rare eye malignancy called retinoblastoma, and polyps of the colon that become malignant. It's possible that heredity may have a part in the more common forms of cancer, too. For example, inherited abnormalities of tissues at certain sites could make them more susceptible to cancerous changes. Also, the growth rates of some cancers are known to be influenced by hormones. Breast cancer in women before menopause may be slowed by male sex hormones, and male cancer of the prostate may be slowed by female sex hormones. So perhaps inherited patterns of hormone secretion are involved in predisposition toward cancer.

Studies of families in which malignancies have appeared indicate that when one member develops a cancer, that same type of cancer occurs more often in that family than in the general population. This has been noted in breast cancer, prostate cancer, and cancers of the stomach and intestines.

But a family history of cancer does not doom one to the disease. Even when there is a demonstrated familial predisposition toward some type of cancer, the risk of developing it may not be overwhelmingly greater for close family members than for other people. For example, where the average woman has a 100-to-1 chance of developing breast cancer, if a woman's mother or sister has had such cancer, the risk is 1 in 50, twice as great as for the average woman. Still, even for her, the chances are 50 to 1 against developing the disease.

Differences in the incidence of various types of cancer in different ethnic and racial groups have been reported. In one study, for example, Polish-born women in the United States were found to have a rate of stomach cancer almost 3 times that of other foreign-born women; colon cancer occurs in Italian-born men 2.7 times more frequently than other foreign-born men;

German-American men had only two-thirds the rate of mouth cancer than did other foreign-born. These differences could well be the result of environmental influences. Some differences have, in fact, been traced to such influences. In Egypt bladder cancer is unusually common, with evidence that a particular parasite found there is responsible. In China liver cancer is unusually common and has been linked with a parasite whose eggs irritate liver cells.

What's the connection between heredity and diabetes?

In diabetes, the body cannot properly utilize carbohydrates because of a lack of sufficient insulin (a hormone produced in the pancreas) or because the insulin is ineffective.

The disease apparently results from the effects of a pair of recessive genes. The inherited factor may be one that causes faulty functioning of pancreas cells and release of inadequate or imperfect insulin. Or it may be a factor leading to body system faults that do not allow the body's insulin to function effectively. It is estimated that about one in four people carry the recessive gene for diabetes.

Even so, environmental factors are important and may govern time of onset and severity. Many persons with unfavorable hereditary predisposition may never develop diabetes, or may develop only a mild form late in life.

Diabetes can be precipitated by obesity, surgery, and pregnancy. It is one of the few major diseases to which women are more vulnerable than men; they have a one-third higher death rate from it.

What about obesity—is that inherited?

There is some evidence that some people gain weight more easily than others and that this tendency may run in families.

As the nutritionist Dr. Jean Mayer has observed: "Farmers have recognized and utilized the genetic determinants of obesity for thousands of years. When animal fat is desired, certain strains predisposed to adiposity are selected in preference to other strains. Plumper pullets and porkers and fatter steers have been bred in this way."

In one study among high school students, fewer than 10 percent of those with parents of normal weight were found to be obese, but 40 percent of those with one obese parent were overweight. If both parents were obese, 80 percent of their children were overweight.

But investigators point out that if fat children tend to have fat parents, family eating habits could be involved. So obesity could be the result of an inherited predisposition, the result of indoctrination, or a combination of both. Some supporting evidence for the possibility of inherited predisposition in humans comes from findings that identical twins tend to be more alike with regard to body weight than do fraternal twins.

Is high blood pressure inherited?

There's no known gene for hypertension, but there is a family predisposition. Many studies have shown that prevalence is greater among close relatives of hypertensive patients than among relatives of normotensives. In one study, for example, the group with the highest prevalence (20.7 percent) consisted of daughters of two hypertensive parents. When only one parent was hypertensive, 13 percent of the daughters had elevated blood pressure. Only 4.5% of the daughters of two normotensive parents had hypertension. Corresponding figures for sons—11 percent, 10 percent, and 7.9 percent respectively—showed a less pronounced effect of family predisposition.

One way in which heredity may influence development of hypertension is through an effect on the way the body handles salt and water. Blood pressure is related to salt and water levels; in fact, hypertension sometimes can be treated successfully by reduction of salt in the diet or by use of diuretic drugs, which help to eliminate excess fluid.

Is there any likelihood that heredity plays a role in infectious diseases?

Certainly there are no genes for pneumonia or influenza or any other infectious disease. Germs are involved. But some people are more susceptible than others. They may have an inherited weakness or lack of resistance that makes them easier prey.

Once, for example, it was thought that tuberculosis was hereditary. But it is now known that TB is caused by infection with a particular germ, the tubercule bacillus. Probably a fair percentage of the population runs a chance of infection. But mere contact with this bacillus is not necessarily enough to produce the infection. The way TB sometimes seems to run in families suggests that resistance to it may be controlled by heredity. Studies have shown that identical twins have a higher risk of being affected simultaneously by tuberculosis—often in the same site or part of the lung—than do nonidentical twins or brothers and sisters, a point in favor of hereditary susceptibility.

But this doesn't mean that a child is born with genes that make TB inevitable. He may have high susceptibility yet remain free of the disease throughout his life if unnecessary risks of infection are avoided.

Are there other diseases influenced by heredity?

Some diseases or disorders show clear-cut hereditary influences. Women carry the gene for hemophilia, but the disease appears only in male descendants. Color blindness is also transmitted by women and appears mostly in men. Glaucoma, a leading cause of blindness, tends to run in families. Family patterns also are known for arthritis.

New hereditary diseases are constantly being discovered—along with ways to control some of them. For example, phenylketonuria (PKU), results from an inherited lack of an enzyme, which can produce mental retardation. PKU is relatively rare, but tests for it are now made routinely at many hospitals; when PKU is discovered, it can be treated effectively by a special diet. Another condition, galactosemia, which involves inability to utilize an ingredient in milk, also results from the absence of an enzyme. It, too, can be discovered by a simple test and treated by diet.

Actually, many discoveries about the influence of heredity in disease have come only in very recent years as the result of more basic knowledge about chromosomes, genes, and genetic behavior.

It is now known that except for a relatively few diseases, mostly rare ones, it is not a matter of only one gene at work.

While physicians long have known of conditions that run in families—conditions ranging from cleft palate to heart ailments, schizophrenia, and rheumatoid arthritis—the familial element has been elusive. Pedigree studies show that none of these conditions is inherited in simple single-gene fashion. Now some idea of what is involved is emerging. Before we can get to that, we have to find out about the basic genetic mechanisms.

Where do genetic mechanisms start?

In a roundish lump of material inside every cell. This is the nucleus—cell headquarters—where cell activities are controlled.

When a cell splits in two for growth or replacement, the nucleus also divides. But it doesn't just split into two equal portions.

It first sorts out into a number of rods, called chromosomes, made of the nucleus material. The nucleus of every body cell of every animal of the same type has the same collection of chromosomes. In human cells there are 46; in guinea pig cells, 62; in crayfish cells, 200; in potato cells (plants have them, too), 48.

As a cell is about to divide, the chromosomes appear not just as single rods but as double ones, each with its two halves lying close together like a pair of sticks placed against each other. During cell division the chromosome halves come unstuck, move away from each other, and sort themselves out into two groups, each made up of an identical set of half chromosomes. The cell divides in a line running between the two chromosome groups, and so the original cell and the new split-off cell each contain a set of half chromosomes. In both mother and daughter cells, the chromosomes soon fuse and form nuclei, and the chromosome material doubles itself before the next cell division takes place. So, for the next division, each cell has its full complement of double chromosomes.

This pattern of cell division holds for all cells as the organism grows, develops, and lives. But when cell division takes place in the cells from which egg or sperm are going to be derived, there are a few differences. The nucleus breaks down as usual into chromosomes—but the chromosomes do not separate into halves. Instead of getting 46 chromosomes (in man), the new egg or sperm cell gets 23. When egg and sperm meet at fertilization, the original number of chromosomes is restored, with half coming from the female and half from the male.

Each chromosome contains thousands of genes, beadlike sections lined up in regular order that is always repeated. They're the hereditary factors, and each is concerned with one or more details of development. While genes can't be seen, infinitely patient research with animals having broken or tangled chromosomes has enabled scientists to draw maps of the chromosomes and show the location of genes that control specific traits.

A gene can be thought of as sending out code messages to the cell, messages about chemicals to be manufactured and what is to be done with them.

Since a child receives one of each pair of chromosomes from the father and the other from the mother, and the genes are laid out along the chromosomes in regular order, the child receives two genes controlling each characteristic. Often the two genes are identical and influence development in the same way. In other instances they differ and may each try to control a particular aspect of development in a different way.

Often, when two genes oppose each other, one is dominant

and can suppress the effects of the other, which is thus called recessive. If a child receives a gene for blue eyes from one parent and a gene for brown eyes from the other, he does not develop bluish brown eyes; instead, he has brown eyes. The gene for brown eyes is dominant.

Astounding as it may seem, the combinations and permutations that may occur in the production of eggs in a woman's ovaries can result in an egg being any one of 8,388,608 different types. And there is similar variety in types of sperms. So the possible number of totally different children that might be produced by a single marriage is at least 70,368,744,177,664. Which, of course, is why brothers and sisters, unless they are identical twins with identical sets of genes, are never exactly alike, since the chances of their getting the same gene assortment are more than 70 million million against.

These odds explain the birth of geniuses to parents of no unusual ability. It's been said—and it's no exaggeration—that within the chromosomes of every man and woman lies the chance to produce a Shakespeare, a Beethoven, an Einstein, or a Lincoln.

What about sex determination?

Among the 46 human chromosomes are two chromosomes that determine sex—one called X, the other Y. In every cell of a female, there are two X chromosomes; in a male, one X and one Y. Every egg the mother produces will, therefore, have an X. But a man produces two kinds of sperm—half containing an X and half containing a Y chromosome. If it's an X-containing sperm that fertilizes the egg, a female child results. If a Y sperm gets to home base first, a boy results.

Genes are called "limit-setters." How come?
What does that mean?

Genes set the bounds, or outer limits, for development. But they don't necessarily determine that the limit will be reached. For example, while genes establish a limit to how tall an individual may grow, other factors determine how tall he actually becomes. In most advanced countries, because of better food, sanitation, and medical care, today's children are usually taller than parents. Similarly, plants living in good soil with suitable amounts of rain and sunshine grow taller than plants growing under less propitious conditions.

The Bach family over the course of three centuries produced twenty members who were composers or musicians. Obviously, genes gave them the edge in talents, but if there had been no family interest in music it's not likely they would have been so successful.

Are attitudes, beliefs, and the like influenced by heredity?

Put it this way: intelligence, reaction speed, motor skills, and sensory discrimination are basic abilities that heredity is most likely to influence. It is *least* likely to have any great effect on beliefs, attitudes, values, and other characteristics that are significantly influenced by training or conditioning. In the middle, some investigators believe, are temperamental traits, such as emotionality, changeability of mood, and activity level.

How do defective genes arise?

By mutation, which means that a gene is changed in some way by some cause. It retains its original position on the chromosome, and when the chromosome is copied during cell division, the gene is reproduced in its new and changed form. A mutated gene can be dominant or recessive, but is most likely to be recessive.

One example of mutation is the albino gene. Skin coloring and hair coloring are controlled by several genes. But there is one gene that provides a chemical used in forming pigments. If it has mutated into an ineffective form, called the albino gene, a crucial part of the coloring process can't occur and the individual will be an albino.

The albino gene is recessive. If a baby has one albino and one normal-coloring gene, he will have normal coloring. For a child to become an albino, he must have the albino gene on both chromosomes of the pair, as the result of mating of two people who have a single albino gene each. Only about 1 in 25,000 times does this happen.

Why do mutations occur at all?

Mutation is a random process. We don't know when or where it's going to happen. It can be a harmful, even lethal mutation; sometimes it's beneficial; frequently, it's neutral.

If it's harmful, those who carry the gene may have a reduced chance or no chance of surviving to reproduce and thereby transmit it. If so, the mutant gene will disappear or will be maintained in the population at very low frequency.

If the mutant produces a change that is not important for survival of those who carry it, it may be lost or stay at low frequency or increase in frequency by pure chance. If it gives a person some important advantage, it is likely to increase in frequency in successive generations until it replaces the original gene.

Are there any examples of helpful mutations?

There's the seemingly strange case of sickle-cell anemia, which occurs mainly among black people and which is now a disease of concern. But when it originated as a mutation in Africa, the gene for sickle-cell anemia represented a successful adaptation to the environment.

The disease arose in malarial regions. It gets its name from the peculiar crescent shape of the red blood cells of an afflicted person. The organism that causes malaria can enter the normal red blood cells but cannot enter sickled cells. So individuals with a mild case of sickle-cell anemia—those who had inherited a single sickle-cell gene—had an advantage in having greater resistance to malaria. But if they inherited two sickle-cell genes, they could die of severe anemia before adolescence.

In some areas of Africa, 40 percent of the population are sickle-cell gene carriers. In areas where the gene serves no useful purpose, it tends to disappear. In the United States, where there is little malaria, sickle-cell gene inheritance is still a problem among blacks but is declining.

Does everyone carry defective genes?

Actually, mutant genes may arise without warning in any generation. Every one of us, according to Dr. Kurt Hirschorn of Mount Sinai Medical School, in New York City, may be carrying from three to eight deleterious genes. However, they are recessive and will not make their presence known unless they combine with similarly defective genes at conception and a child is born with a defect.

Pellagra is an example of a vitamin deficiency disease that originated through gene mutation, perhaps millions of years ago, and was cured by eating other organisms that do manufacture the antipellagra vitamin man no longer produces because of the mutation. (Of course, our ancestors didn't know what precisely they were doing. They stumbled on cures by chance and natural selection preserved the new habit.) Gene mutations produced diseases in our ancestors for each vitamin we now require. We keep such diseases under control by eating as a matter of habit what is called a proper diet.

Abraham Lincoln may have had a genetically induced disturbance called Marfan's syndrome. It involves a disorder of connective tissue. Only in 1959 did a California physician, Dr. Harold Schwartz, first suspect Lincoln's problem when he diagnosed it in a seven-year-old boy, who turned out to share ancestry with Lincoln. Like Lincoln, the boy was unusually long-limbed, which is one indication of the disorder. Marfan's syndrome also includes asymmetries in the body and, frequently, eye trouble. Lincoln not only had unusually long arms and legs but marked disproportions between right and left sides, plus eye trouble—severe farsightedness and difficulty in coordinating his eyes.

How are genetic problems forecast?

It's possible not so much to forecast but to calculate odds on whether a couple may have a defective child, if genetic defects can be traced back through family trees.

Some diseases can be produced by a single dominant defective gene. Achondroplasia, a type of dwarfism, is caused by such a dominant gene, and any child inheriting the gene will have the disease. A genetic counselor could warn a parent who has such a disease that half of his children risk having it.

More often, recessive genes are responsible for hereditary disorders. An example is cystic fibrosis, which affects about one in 1,600 babies, causing their lungs and other body organs to become congested with mucus. A child inheriting one recessive gene for cystic fibrosis will be a carrier but will not have the disease. If both parents are carriers of the gene, one in four of their children will have the disease, two will be carriers, and one will be normal.

Some diseases such as hemophilia are sex-linked recessive gene defects. The defective gene is carried on the female X-chromosome. The disease is produced only in male children when the X chromosome bearing the faulty gene pairs with the father's Y chromosome. Half the sons of a female hemophiliac carrier will risk the disease; half the daughters may be carriers.

In order for a female child to get a sex-linked disease, the father must have the disease and the mother must be a carrier. The mother's defective X chromosome pairs with the defective X chromosome of the father, and the female child will have the disease. However, this is rare.

In recent years several disorders caused by an extra chromosome, or the lack of part of a chromosome, have been detected. Mongolism, a form of retardation accompanied by short stature, flattened nose, and broad hands and feet, is produced by an extra chromosome. Parents who have had one such child have little increased risk of having another mongolian, but in a few cases the mongolism can be passed on from generation to generation by carriers. One in three of a carrier's children is likely to be mongolian; one, a carrier; and one, normal.

But isn't genetic counseling become more scientific?

There have been significant recent advances. Previously counseling had to rely largely on estimates based on the law of averages. But investigators have begun to develop laboratory tests to detect carriers. Blood, urine, and other tests show promise for detecting carriers of more than 100 genetic diseases, including cystic fibrosis, PKU, hemophilia, and some forms of muscular dystrophy. Consequently, a genetic counselor now can tell with reasonable certainty whether the sister of a man with hemophilia is a carrier.

It's now possible to check chromosomes for defects; if certain chromosomal abnormalities are found, the prospective parents can be told that they almost certainly will have deformed offspring. If such knowledge takes some of the mystery and romance out of procreation, it also eliminates some of the uncertainty and dread. As one geneticist observes, "There is nothing very romantic about a mongoloid child or a deformed body."

An even more important advance is amniocentesis, which is a technique by which the cells of the unborn early in development can be studied to establish with accuracy whether the infant will inherit his parents' defective genes.

Amniocentesis (from the Greek *amnion*, meaning membrane, and *kentesis*, meaning pricking) is performed by inserting a long needle through the mother's abdomen and into her uterus to draw off a small sample of amniotic fluid, the amber liquid in which the fetus floats. The fetal cells are separated from the fluid and placed in a nutrient bath where they continue to grow and divide. By microscopic examination and chemical analysis, any of nearly seventy different genetic disorders can be identified.

Amniocentesis is relatively safe, but not 100 percent free of risk. But where family history indicates the possibility of genetic defects, the benefits of the tests may more than justify the risks.

In a typical case, a pregnant woman was known to be carrying the extra chromosome responsible for mongolism. Amniocentesis settled the question about her unborn child; the child would be a mongolian idiot. The woman had a therapeutic abortion. Some months later, when she was pregnant again, amniocentesis was repeated and this time the fetal cell study showed the child would be normal. It was normal.

In addition to prenatal diagnosis, prenatal treatment of some conditions is now possible. Physicians routinely carry out intrauterine transfusions of blood on fetuses when the mother has Rh-negative blood and is incompatible with the fetal blood.

Thus far, medical genetics has been most successful in illuminating the relatively rare hereditary diseases, those produced by a single gene and whose transmission can be traced in families with relative ease.

What about predicting the more common defects?

Many of the more common diseases seem to be partially genetic. They are familial, but they don't involve a particular defective gene. Instead they appear to be the result of the interaction of an unknown number of genes with many environmental factors. Diabetes, rheumatoid arthritis, and even schizophrenia are believed to involve genetic factors. But they seem to be triggered by environmental influences, and the part played by genes is difficult to establish.

Guilt can be assigned by association—by establishing that a particular disease is more common in certain families than in the general population or that identical twins suffer from it more often than do nonidentical twins.

For example, diabetes runs in families. If one identical twin has it, there is a 62 percent chance that the other will have it, too. Clearly, powerful genetic influences are at work. But it is also clear that genes can't be the whole story; otherwise either both twins or neither would be affected.

Cleft palate is another example. If one identical twin has it, the other will be affected only four times out of ten. That's about four hundred times the chance expectation in the general population. Genes are involved, but so is something else.

What's the answer? A heredity-environment tug-of-war?

It now seems that familial disorders are multifactorial, meaning that each involves a sizable number of different hereditary and environmental influences.

Their heredity component is polygenic, reflecting the activity of many genes rather than one. Since many genes are involved, there is not a fixed genetic predisposition to a disease as there would be if just one gene mattered. Instead, there is a range of genetic predisposition—a little, a moderate amount, a lot. And the actual development of a disease requires that the genetic predisposition be strong enough to push the individual up to a point of risk—at which point environmental influences will determine whether, and sometimes to what extent, he will be affected.

It seems complex—and it is. But many of the most basic and obvious human characteristics, such as height and body build, are multifactorially determined. These traits vary across a fairly wide range: there are people seven feet tall and people five feet tall. But most people have midrange values.

Any time there is such a distribution over a range, there is strong evidence of multifactorial influence. An analogy can be made to flipping coins. Flip a single coin and it has to come up heads or tails. That's a single or monofactorial situation. It's analogous to a condition determined by just a single gene. But now flip, say, six coins. You might get three heads and three tails, but you could also get a range of other combinations. That's a multifactorial situation.

What does it all mean?

That while heredity is responsible for some serious diseases, they are the rare kinds. Heredity usually acts as a factor that may predispose the body toward the disease, but does not make the disease inevitable. Although you can't control your heredity, you do have control over many, even most, of the other risk factors for diseases.

For example, a hereditary predisposition toward atherosclerosis doesn't inevitably mean fat-clogged arteries and heart attack if other factors—blood pressure, weight, blood fats, and still others—don't enhance the predisposition. Keep such risk factors under beneficent control and you can relax about family predisposition; it's not enough in itself to hurt you.

Look at it another way, too. You can take advantage of your

knowledge. If your forebears died early of heart attacks, you have an edge in knowing the significance of family tendency and what the other risk factors are and the value of controlling them. Fatalism is no longer in order. *You can protect yourself.*

3

Male versus Female

How much of an edge on longevity do women have?

Unless some way is found to help men live longer, women may take over the country. There are some 5.5 million more women than men in the United States. After age twenty-five, women outnumber men in all age groups. For every 1,000 men over sixty-five, there are 1,276 women. Two-thirds of all married women in the country are widows by age sixty-five. Widows outnumber widowers 3 to 1. The life expectancy at birth for girls is about seven years longer than for boys.

Even beginning in the womb there are 50 percent fewer deaths for female fetuses. There are more deaths for males among premature babies, and in the first year of life the death rate is about 25 percent higher for males.

From ages five to nine, male deaths are about 20 percent higher; from ten to fourteen, about 40 percent. From fifteen to nineteen almost three times as many males die as females. Deaths of males in the late twenties exceed those of females by 2 to 1. Between the years thirty-five and thirty-nine, the male death rate is 3 per 1,000 population while the female is 1.9. In the early forties, it's 4.6 for men, 2.8 for women; and in the late forties, 7.5 versus 4.2.

And that's the way it keeps going. The death rate per 1,000 in the late fifties is 19 for men, 9.4 for women; in the early sixties, 28.2 for men, 14.5 for women; in the late sixties 43.6 versus 22.8; and in the seventies, 60.5 versus 35.7.

It appears that not only in humans but in all living species—and this has been observed in mice, rats, guinea pigs, and others—the female is longer-lived. Which suggests that, biologically, the female may be the stronger sex.

Are women more resistant to all diseases?

Not to all, but to many of the most important diseases. Women are much more resistant to heart disease, which is the number one killer. According to various surveys, men are five to twenty times more vulnerable to coronaries during middle age than women are. In the government's Framingham study, which began in 1949 and has been following more than 5,000 people in that Massachusetts community ever since, no woman under age forty experienced a heart attack; on the average, in Framingham, women are ten to twenty years older than men when they do get heart attacks.

At ages forty-five to fifty-four, the annual cardiovascular disease rate for men is close to three times as great as for women; at ages fifty-five to sixty-four, it's two and a half times as great; even at ages sixty-five to seventy-four, it's almost twice as great.

Cancer seems to have little regard for sex. For most cancers, the risk is slightly greater for women until age sixty-five, and thereafter is about equal between the sexes. But lung cancer strikes four and a half times as many males as females. Overall, the chances at birth of eventually dying from cancer are 162 per 1,000 for males, 155 for females.

For both men and women, the chances of dying from pneumonia and influenza are about the same—approximately 33 per 1,000. Tuberculosis is now a relatively minor cause of death; the present chances of dying from it are less than 5 per 1,000 for males, no more than 2 per 1,000 for females.

Diabetes is one of the few causes of death for which women have a substantially higher risk. The chances at birth of eventual death from diabetes are 24 per 1,000 for women compared with 14 for men.

Accidents rank well up among leading threats to life. Here again women do better. The chances at birth for men to eventually die of an accident are 61 per 1,000; for women, 36 per 1,000. The chances diminish with age but are still at least 25 per 1,000 for both men and women at age sixty-five. The greater death rate for men before mid-life in large part results from their more frequent involvement in motor vehicle accidents. After sixty-five, other forms of accidents are a more serious threat to women than to men.

Is it a matter of hormones?

The female of the species may be endowed from the first moment of life with a body chemistry that gives her more life-prolonging materials. And that includes sex hormones. Women and men produce both female hormones, called estrogen, and male hormones, called androgens. In women there are more estrogens than androgens; in men, the opposite.

The female hormone, estrogen, lowers the fat content of the blood. It appears therefore to provide a significant degree of protection against coronary atherosclerosis, in which the coronary arteries that feed the heart become clogged with fat. Before menopause, women are relatively immune to coronary disease and the sequel, heart attack. This immunity is a major factor in their great longevity.

Millions of American women past menopause now take estrogen tablets as a means of overcoming the consequences of change of life. The pills are used to keep the breasts firm, the bones hard, the muscles and skin well-toned. Do they also help guard against coronary attacks? Some physicians think they may; others dispute the idea.

Judging from animal experiments reported in 1971 by Dr. Grace M. Fischer of the University of Pennsylvania, female arteries have more flexibility than do male arteries. Estrogen seems to help keep arteries from becoming stiff and unstretchable, and their greater flexibility may help offset the artery hardening and fat clogging that set the stage for heart attacks.

An artery wall is composed of large amounts of connective tissue, the structural material that serves as supporting framework for body organs. Connective tissue itself is made up chiefly of two kinds of fibers, collagen and elastin. Collagen is the tougher, more rigid element. Working with female rats whose ovaries had been removed and hence lacked normal amounts of estrogen, Dr. Fischer found that the rats given supplemental injections of estrogen had a higher proportion of the more stretchable elastin fibers and therefore their arteries were less stiff than those of the rats not given estrogen.

What's wrong with male hormones?

Nothing, when it comes to beards, muscular strength, virility, and the like. But they seem in some way to stimulate, rather than counter, certain disease factors.

Those docile harem slaves in the *Arabian Nights* who never

won the ladies' favors may have outlived the sultan. Castrated males live longer than intact ones, according to a recent study by Dr. James B. Hamilton and a team from the State University of New York Downstate Medical Center, Brooklyn. The study covered 297 eunuchs and 735 intact males in an institution for the mentally retarded. Hamilton was dealing with a study group castrated decades ago; no mental institution today is known to practice castration. The men were matched for age, length of institutionalization, and physical condition.

The average life-span for the eunuchs was found to be 69.3 years; for the intact males, 55.7 Moreover, those castrated before reaching the age of fourteen lived substantially longer than those castrated after twenty. Hamilton also observed that castrated males even outlived intact females.

Is there any genetic advantage conferred by sex?

There is a theory that the key to female superiority lies in the sex determination mechanism that parcels out more genes to women than to men.

As noted earlier, a child's sex depends entirely upon which of the 200 million sperm in an ejaculation wins the race to fertilize the egg. Recall that women have two X sex chromosomes, men have one X and one Y, and that each sex cell—egg or sperm—has half the complement of sex chromosomes. Therefore an egg always has an X but a sperm can have either an X or a Y. If an X-bearing sperm fertilizes the egg, it's an X-plus-X matter and the child is girl. If a Y-bearer does the fertilizing, it's X-plus-Y and the child is a boy. (The Y-bearers apparently have a slightly better chance of doing the fertilizing; 106 boys are born for every 100 girls.)

Now the fact is that the two types of sex chromosomes, X and Y, are an oddly assorted pair. The X is one of the largest of all chromosomes in the cell. It's about three times the size of the Y and is apparently far more active in body functioning. It contains many more genes.

It's generally believed that while the X chromosome has undergone little change in the course of evolution, the Y has grown progressively smaller and less influential as mammals have evolved—and, as of now, its only established role is as a determiner of sex.

Thus one might say that every male is shortchanged at birth. He has fewer genes than the female with her two X chromosomes—on the order of 500 to 1,000 fewer.

If one or more genes on his X chromosome are not up to par, he has no spares on his Y chromosome to offset them. If a girl has a bad X gene, the chances are good that the other X chromosome will carry a normal gene and the effects of the bad gene will be inhibited. But if a boy has a bad X gene it may produce a disease or defect. Hemophilia, for instance, almost never strikes females because they have additional normal genes on their second X chromosome. And color blindness is eight times as frequent in boys as in girls.

Could the male Y chromosome in itself be a baleful influence?

That's a possibility that is being explored by Dr. James B. Hamilton. The latest work of Hamilton and his group, reported in 1970, suggests that even if androgen is eliminated, the Y chromosome in itself may somehow reduce viability.

The researchers have studied the sex chromosome effect for eight years in little striped minnows called killifish. They find that if hatchling killifish are fed estrogen before their sex glands mature, XY females can be produced. And when these unusual females are mated with normal XY males, one-fourth of the next hatch of hatchlings are YY males. If the YYs are fed estrogen, they become YY females. So, by breeding YY males with YY females, all the YY males needed for the experiments could be turned out.

Whereas normal XY male killifish have a median life span of 501 days, Hamilton found that the life-span of YYs was only 415 days. And, significantly, there were greater losses among the YY supermales in the first three weeks of life, before the gonads matured and therefore before androgen might play any deleterious role.

Hamilton is planning to study the life-span of YY killifish whose gonads have been removed as another check on the relationship of the Y chromosome to survival. He hopes that some day it may be possible to lengthen the life-span of men without making them pay a penalty in virility. Hamilton, one medical magazine observes, is a "warrior in the cause of equal biological rights for man."

Hormone-chromosome theories aside, don't men have a tougher life, and doesn't that account for their shorter lives?

Those who favor this idea say that women live longer than men because men wear themselves out working for women. But those who oppose the idea point to a recent study made by two sociologists, the Reverend Francis Madigan, a Jesuit priest, and Rupert Vance of the University of North Carolina of the comparative life expectancies of 42,000 Catholic nuns and brothers. All were white, native-born, unmarried teachers, all living the same type of life free from many of the stresses and financial cares common to laymen. The study found that the life expectancy of nuns was 5.5 years greater than that of the brothers, suggesting that the longevity advantage enjoyed by women could be more biological than environmental.

Of course, many investigators still wonder about tensions in the male. Does he meet greater stress in his work than the woman does in the home, even considering the frustrations a wife and mother may encounter?

What other factors may favor women?

Some heart experts suggest that women make more effort, because of fashion, to avoid obesity. While the eating habits of men and women tend to be similar, women may eat somewhat less or avoid more of the richer foods. Generally, American women are less overweight than men, and they are slimmer than they were at the turn of the century. On the other hand, men today are fatter than they were forty or fifty years ago, and they generally eat foods higher in calories, cholesterol, and total fats, all of which are implicated in heart disease.

Of course, machines have been a great boon to women. But women are still active—especially women who hold down several jobs as housewife, mother, and employee. Women generally may have a more healthful level of daily activity; even with labor-saving devices in the home, they may move about a lot more than men, whose jobs tend to be increasingly sedentary.

Women are credited with being more careful of their health, with taking better care of themselves when sick, and with seeking earlier treatment of illness. Women may be ill more often than men, but they are not as often seriously ill. One study found that men are absent from work because of disabling illness twice as much during the ages forty-five through sixty-four as are women workers of those ages.

What about behavioral differences between the sexes?
Do they count?

Some conceivably may influence health and longevity. Such differences show up early in life. Boy infants generally sleep less

than girls, cry more, demand more attention. Female babies tend
to be more passive, to smile more often, and seemingly to learn
more rapidly.

Some psychologists point out that at age twelve weeks, girls
look longer at pictures of faces than at geometrical figures. Boys
show no preferences at twelve weeks, but later tend to prefer the
geometrical form. Such studies suggest that even early in life
females express preferences they will develop more fully later on.
Generally, the psychologists say, girls find satisfactions in relating with people to a greater extent than do boys. They learn
to talk earlier and more fluently, are more docile, strive harder
to please both at home and in school. Later, they tend to choose
work—such as teaching, nursing, child care, social service—that
usually involves close interaction with people.

If psychological studies are right, women are, much more than
men, influenced by the opinions and feelings of others. They
attach more importance to encouragement and praise—more
even than to a prospect of promotion. In fact, according to some
investigators, one career problem for women may be that as they
climb up the ladder they may reach levels where praise is rare
and competition keener.

In contrast, boys tend to be quarrelsome, to give teachers more
trouble, to get lower grades through high school, and to maintain
a greater interest in things rather than in people. Men, it appears, are stimulated by competition, and work not only for
money but for power and to win over others. No matter how high
they go men tend to be less content with their achievements than
women do.

What causes these differences, nature or nurture?

The current idea is that behavioral patterns result from a
complex interaction between inheritance and environment—nature and nurture. But for a long time people assumed that the
two sexes inherited differences in temperament much as they
did those in body. Men were supposed to be superior. Then, about
the turn of the century, as coeducation began to develop and
women began to demand equal rights and invaded some traditional male fields, the innate difference idea lost ground rapidly.
Environment was the thing.

Dr. Frank Beach of the University of California, who had his
training in the early 1930s, recalls, "At that time the psychologists were all environmentalists, and it was simply unthinkable

to say that the sexes could differ psychologically for any reason except conditioning. Nobody argued that a woman's size, general body formation, or reproductive anatomy were not strongly influenced by genetic factors.

"But the curtain dropped when it got to psychology, as through the brain, which controls behavior, was unaffected. I can recall getting scolded when I even raised the issue, because if you said that boys and girls differed, it seemed automatically to mean that one was inferior and the other superior.

"Even then tests were coming out showing that boys did better in math and girls in English, but if you suggested this kind of thing had genetic origins at all it somehow suggested that girls were inferior. Why English should be inferior to math, I don't know."

What's the prevailing opinion today?

On the psychological side, a popular concept is that role modeling has much to do with personality differences between the sexes. At about eighteen months of age, a child begins to identify itself as either male or female, and then looks around for, and picks up, clues as to what his or her personality should be.

Obviously, role modeling helps shape personality and behavior. Anthropologists studying many different cultures have found that in at least half of them women, not men, do virtually all the heavy work. Much of the commerce in some societies, particularly in West Africa, is female-controlled. In the Soviet Union, unlike the United States, medicine is largely a woman's profession: three-fourths of Russian doctors are women.

But role modeling is not the whole answer. As one critic puts it, role modeling, as a total explanation for behavioral and personality differences between the sexes, "faces certain logical difficulties."

One problem is that some traits—male aggressiveness, for example—are displayed very early, presumably before the child knows which parent to model after. "Similarly, it seems unlikely that, for example, male children are able to discern subtle differences in their parents' intellectual styles by the early age at which males begin to evidence signs of their superiority at spatial reasoning. So, while males and females need to respond to their culture's peculiar orchestration, they hear the beat of inner drums as well."

What's faulty with Women's Lib ideas about sex differences?

A refusal to recognize that those "inner drums" exist—an attempt to minimize any inherent differences between the sexes—strikes some researchers as one of the least acceptable aspects of Women's Lib. "The main thrust of their debate, or more correctly their assertions, is that such differences as exist are merely the result of differences in education and training, and therefore not basic. . . . But in fact the sexes differ so markedly in ways that are not subject to change—anatomy and physiology—that it is a serious mistake to ignore them or try to make them disappear by talking," says Dr. Paul Popenoe.

Popenoe points out the following facts:

1. Men and women differ in every body cell because of sex chromosome combination.

2. Women have greater constitutional vitality, possibly beuse of the chromosomal difference.

3. Basal metabolism—the base rate at which body processes take place and energy is produced—differs between the sexes, that of women being normally lower than that of men.

4. Skeletal structure differs, with women having shorter heads, broader faces, less protruding chins, shorter legs, and longer trunks.

5. Women have bodily functions—menstruation, pregnancy, lactation—not present in men, and they influence behavior and feelings.

6. The thyroid gland in women behaves differently than in men. It is larger, more active, and enlarges during menstruation and pregnancy, making for increased proneness to goiter but also more resistance to temperature changes. It is associated with smoother skin, relatively hairless body, a layer of subcutaneous fat that provides feminine curves; its activity also contributes to emotional instability and women tend to laugh and cry more easily.

7. In women's blood there is more water but 20 percent fewer red cells. Since it is the hemoglobin in red cells that supplies oxygen to the body, women having less of it tire more easily than men and faint more readily. An example of how this perfectly normal biological functioning in women affects their place in industry is to be found in British factories during World War II when, under pressure to produce more, the working day was increased to twelve hours. There was a 150 percent increase in accidents among women workers, none among men.

Aren't sex hormones involved in behavior?

Apparently they have much more influence than was previously thought. The prevailing idea had been that up to puberty, male and female sex hormones are present in equal amounts in girls and boys alike. The idea gave support to the role-modeling concept that learning must account for differences in behavior between the sexes.

Then, about 20 years ago, animal studies began to indicate that prior to birth some aspects of behavioral as well as anatomical differences between the sexes were determined. When researchers injected small amounts of male hormone into female guinea pigs before birth, lasting changes occurred in behavior as well as anatomy. Female by inheritance, the pigs developed male sex organs and male mating behavior. When repeated with animals more closely related to man, the experiments brought the same results.

In man and all mammals, it appears, bodies and brains are organized not male first and female second, but vice versa. Every human fetus is predisposed to develop into a female, *unless* a special event occurs. That special event—triggered by the presence of the male sex chromosome—is a temporary upsurge in androgen production by the fetal sex organs. The upsurge sets up a chain of events that leads to maleness. Maleness in body, it's believed, is accompanied by maleness in brain, a kind of patterning of brain circuits for maleness.

The female circuits are obliterated during the change toward maleness. They appear to continue functioning to some extent and may make some contributions to male behavior throughout life. In animal experiments, researchers have been able to show that injections of female hormone at certain brain sites can lead adult males to ape the mating and maternal behavior of females, and vice versa with male hormones in females.

Thus sex hormones are important in determining behavior, because tiny amounts early in development apparently establish some kind of patterning that at least in part helps determine the kinds of experiences and molding the individual is likely to accept or reject.

According to some investigators, influences of sex hormones on the nervous system account for the fact that women generally tend to have more acute senses of hearing, taste, and touch than men do. But such increased sensory perceptiveness may also cause women to feel pain more acutely when hurt, and to want, more than most men, to avoid stressful situations when they can.

*What is the significance of environmental influences
on the difference in longevity between the sexes?*

Environmental influences show up, for example, in the varying death rates for men and women in different countries. While
it's a fact that in the United States heart disease claims about
twice as many men as women between the ages of forty and
seventy-four, it's also true that in other countries the excess of
male deaths ranges widely—from a high of 118 percent in
Australia to only 13 percent in Italy.

It's also noteworthy that the markedly greater life expectancy
of women is a recent phenomenon. Ancient records, and even
those up to about a century ago, give no indication that women
as a general rule outlived men. In the United States and other
advanced countries the margin for women has recently doubled
from the two or three years it was in 1900. In the more backward
countries, the worse the living and health conditions, the smaller
the margin of female over male life expectancy, to the point
where it disappears or male expectancy is even higher. For example, life expectancy in Bolivia is the same for both sexes—
49.7 years. In Guatemala, Ceylon, Cambodia, and Upper Volta
it is higher for men by a few months.

Can these differences be explained?

One explanation is that men are exposed to many special environmental hazards such as jobs, war, higher accident rates,
harder and more careless living. Women, too, run a special risk
during childbirth. But where once, with unrestricted childbearing
and little if any medical attention, childbirth produced heavy
casualties, now the great reduction in childbearing danger (maternal mortality now is less than 1 per 2,000 births) is an environmental plus for women that has countered a natural
disadvantage.

Modern conditions have tended to make life somewhat easier
for women as a group than for men. In the past hardships and
dangers were often shared almost equally by the two sexes. If
women have an inherent advantage for longer life, this advantage might well be limited under unfavorable conditions and
able to show up more in a favorable environment.

Another factor of modern life may deserve consideration, "new
masculinity." Anthropologists such as Dr. Ethel Alpenfels of New
York University consider "new masculinity" to be abroad in the
land in this sense: The frontier era of exploration and rugged

masculinity is gone, and the current tend is to climb up the status ladder to provide for wife and family what other men provide. The pressures are tremendous, says Alpenfels, pointing to her studies with young men who have had heart attacks and pressure-related human problems.

She also observes that if unmarried women with financial burdens don't die as young as men, or have ulcers and heart attacks, it's because they are permitted to show their emotions, whereas from boyhood on, males are taught that it is not masculine to cry. Dr. Aspenfels predicts less emphasis on masculinity and femininity in the future and more on people as people.

What does all this mean in terms of longevity?

From a practical standpoint, women seem to have an innate advantage for long life, everything else being equal. For men, though, the situation is far from hopeless. If men don't have the innate push in the right direction that women have, they still can supply some healthy shoves, because many other factors enter into the health and longevity picture.

4

Childhood and
Early Experience

Can season of birth affect health and longevity?

Some investigators believe that weather influences us from the moment of conception; that the month and season of the year in which we're conceived has a decided effect in determining how healthy and long-lived we're likely to be. They maintain that human fertility has seasonal ups and downs; that in late spring people are at their sexual peak and perhaps their physical peak as well. At this season not only are they most prolific but also their children, if conceived then, are off to a good start.

What does the evidence show?

Dr. Ellsworth Huntington of Yale made studies of millions of births. According to his findings, children conceived in May and June and born in February and March tend to be more intelligent, to become stronger and hardier adults, and to live longer. When, for example, Huntington compared one group of people conceived in June and born in March with another group conceived in October and born in July, he found that on the average the March-born lived 3.8 years longer than the July-born.

A case can also be made for early spring conception. Studying *Who's Who* entries for 80,000 distinguished Americans—industrialists, physicians, scientists, engineers, authors, clergymen, and so on—Huntington found a preponderance of January and

34

February births, suggesting that, at least from the achievement standpoint, early spring conception has its merits.

Apparently, season of birth can also have some influence on infant death rates. Working from recent official tabulations of the National Vital Statistics Division, investigators found that the highest infant mortality rate occurs among those born in May and June.

Some studies suggest an influence on mental illness. In one of the most recent, investigators of the Lafayette Clinic in Detroit checked on 469 emotionally disturbed children at seventeen child treatment centers in the United States and one in Canada, comparing them with several hundred children who did not show emotional disturbances. They found that seriously disturbed children were most likely to have been conceived during the hot months. Some work by the same group, now in progress, suggests tentatively that the IQs of summer-conceived children tend to be lower.

Still another recent study by the New York State Health Department Birth Defects Institute found an unexplained relationship between teeth that do not line up properly and April, May, and June birth dates. The phenomenon first turned up in a random sampling of 1,413 high school students; of those with the dental defect, a disproportionate number were born in one of the three months. A later check of other children with dental defects found a greater than average number born in April, May, and June. Since birth in those months means conception in July, August, or September, there is some speculation that bacterial and viral infections common in summer and early fall might be a cause.

Do cosmic influences have any demonstrable effects?

"If Mars was at its zenith when your baby was born does that mean he might become a great doctor? Of course not. But then on the other hand . . ."

That's the way a news release from the American Medical Association not long ago started off, leading into a discussion of some recent findings that may support the idea. It noted that Michel Gauguelin, an investigator in the field of biomagnetics, which evaluates the effect of the earth's magnetic field on animal life, had found a surprising correlation between the position of the planets at the birth of great men and their eventual occupations. In the course of investigating the lives of 25,000 men from all over Europe, he determined that certain occupations were clustered around specific planets: that eminent doctors showed an unaccountable statistical preference for being born when either Mars or Saturn had just risen or was at its zenith; for actors, it was Jupiter; for writers, the moon.

Gauguelin suggests that the magnetic forces of a heavenly body may act on a particular genetic code, the magnetic force serving as a "releaser" at birth.

Whether or not magnetism plays such a role, other researchers have noticed other effects of biomagnetics. It is known that the composition of human blood can be altered by sunspots; and that psychiatric admissions increase during magnetic storms. In the past five years, investigators have been able to show that a variety of organisms, ranging from birds to insects, respond sensitively to the earth's very weak magnetic field.

The AMA report does note, "Serious investigators in the field are impatient with what they call the 'mystics' of the field of biomagnetics. Scientists feel these people are too eager to assign a wide range of diseases, including mental illness, to sunspots and other disturbances of the magnetic field of the earth. But as the effects of biomagnetics are charted, it becomes more apparent that the field shows a great potential for having profound effects on politics, history, sociology, and medicine."

Does order of birth appear to influence later life?

Recently investigators have reported findings suggesting that many traits may reflect at least to some extent a child's position in his family. The evidence, though, is not always conclusive.

On the average a firstborn weighs less at birth than later children. Within two or three years, he is heavier than his siblings will be when they reach that age. But by adulthood there is no significant difference among them in weight and height.

Other studies indicate that asthma tends to strike firstborn more often than other children; duodenal ulcer, the lastborn; and that by age four later-born have twice as many infections as do firstborn.

The findings about mental illness seem somewhat contradictory. Some studies indicate a slightly greater tendency toward schizophrenia among later-born children, especially girls. Others find that firstborn are referred more often to clinics because of anxiety and severe psychotic symptoms. There is some suggestion, too, that later-born children are more likely to be mentally retarded.

Some psychiatric studies suggest that firstborn are more likely to be introverts and later-born to be extroverts, although there are many striking exceptions among celebrated men and women. Analyses of mothers' reports indicate that they find their first-born likely to be more timid, tense, and fearful than later children. At least one psychological study indicates that firstborn tend to have more extreme fears related to social and interpersonal situations such as being alone and parting from friends.

Later-born seem more disposed toward temper tantrums, bedwetting, and nightmares and more likely to be overactive, negative, destructive, and given to lying. At child guidance centers, firstborn, especially girls, are brought in more often with behavior problems, ranging from school phobia to stealing, but this could be a result of the inexperience and worries of young parents.

It's in the area of intellectual achievement that firstborn, including only children, seem to stand out.

Are firstborn more intelligent?

Of 235 Rhodes scholars from two-child families, 61.3 percent were firstborn. Two out of three finalists in the National Merit Scholarship competitions are firstborn. Among people listed in *Who's Who*, 64 percent are firstborn.

A check of 1,817 college students from two-child families on a University of California campus showed that 63 percent of those who excelled were firstborn. In the scholastically more exacting colleges firstborn enrollment is often much higher than it is in colleges that admit students with lower scholastic standings. For example, at Reed College in Portland, Oregon, 66 percent of a sample were firstborn and at Yale 61 percent, while at a less exacting midwestern state university the figure was about 50 percent.

Firstborn children not infrequently are sensitive introverts, and they may well be creative. There is a predominance of firstborn among great poets, including Byron, Keats, Shelley, Milton, and Shakespeare. Some of the great creative thinkers in other areas, Einstein and Freud, for example, were firstborn children.

A current theory now holds that the sacrifice of firstborn children in the Mediterranean area—not uncommon for several centuries before Christ—may have influenced civilization there to a great extent. In the city of Carthage, for example, firstborn were often sacrificed for religious purposes. Carthaginians left no notable architecture and contributed little to literature, philosophy, or science. It's difficult to prove that this lack of inspiration resulted from sacrificing the firstborn, but some scientists believe it is not unlikely.

A bit discouraging for later-born, isn't it?

Not really. Benjamin Franklin had a number of preceding siblings. John F. Kennedy, Thomas A. Edison, and Dwight D. Eisenhower had older brothers. Firstborn scarcely have a monopoly on superior intelligence or other advantageous traits. Here are two lists to consider.

FIRSTBORN	LATER-BORN
Alexander the Great	Napoleon Bonaparte
Dante Alighieri	Albert Camus
Ludwig van Beethoven	Miguel de Cervantes
Thomas Carlyle	T. S. Eliot
William Faulkner	Benjamin Franklin
Sigmund Freud	Alexander Hamilton
Johann von Goethe	Andrew Jackson
Barry Goldwater	Søren Kierkegaard
Thomas Jefferson	Nikolai Lenin
Lyndon Johnson	Herman Melville
Karl Marx	Friedrich Nietzsche
John Milton	Richard Nixon
Jawaharlal Nehru	Alfred Nobel
Alexander Pope	Jean Jacques Rousseau
Arthur Schopenhauer	Henry David Thoreau
William Shakespeare	Leo Tolstoi
Jonathan Swift	Richard Wagner
George Washington	Walt Whitman

It has been held by sociological theory that firstborn sons tend to be tradition carriers because of greater parental involvement with them, while later sons are tradition breakers and innovators because they get less parental attention, but the list above shows obvious exceptions.

Moreover, so far as achievement is concerned, personality, motivation, hard work, and other factors play significant roles. It has also been observed that even if superior intelligence is a boost, few men use all the intelligence they have, which allows others, who may be less ably endowed, a chance to excel. It also seems that any greater likelihood for firstborn to achieve success may be considerably offset when conditions of high stress enter the picture. Among U.S. fighter pilots in the Korean conflict, firstborn pilots as a group didn't do as well as later-born pilots. The latter were much more likely to achieve "ace" ranking. Among divers in the navy's Project Sealab II, firstborn spent less time than later-born in performing tasks under water outside the Sea-lab capsule, which was classed as stressful environment. Over a fifteen-day period, later-born averaged nearly 77 percent more time outside.

But if firstborn are more fearful in highly stressful situations —and Sealab firstborn owned up to a higher level of fright than others—they also get themselves into these situations more often, overproportionately volunteering for stressful as well as non-stressful challenges. All seven of the original Mercury astronauts were firstborn; twelve of the fifteen candidates for the Gemini program were firstborn or the only male offspring; sixteen of the twenty-eight Sealab aquanauts were firstborn.

Do parental attitudes differ significantly between
firstborn and later-born?

There is a theory that parents tend to instill higher standards in firstborn and reward them more consistently for being parent-oriented. However, firstborn have only their parents as early guides to behavior and achievement, and they find it difficult to emulate them. So firstborn may have higher goals and a greater feeling of connection with the Establishment but lower self-esteem and self-confidence. In addition, when great stress is involved in an achievement task, they tend to be hampered by anxiety.

Parents usually insist that their attitudes toward firstborn and later-born do not differ significantly. But some observers, according to Theodore Irwin writing in an American Medical Association publication, believe that in most families parents "load the dice" for the first child from the beginning. They tend to exaggerate his importance, and to treat him as a companion. Chances are he is planned for and wanted. He is likely to be breast-fed longer. But the parents, since they're young and new to parenthood, may not be sure of themselves and may communicate their anxieties to the child. Mothers often admit that while they were nervous with the first child, they became more relaxed and self-assured with later children.

Restrictions and physical punishment are often harsher with the oldest child, some studies indicate. Easing up with experience, parents may be less inclined to spank youngest children. The age of the parents may be a factor; investigators report that mothers in their thirties appear to be more indulgent, even with firstborn, than younger women are.

A Columbia University experiment seems to indicate that,

even if they don't realize it, parents may tend to make a firstborn or only child more dependent. In the experiment, carried out with sixty four-year-olds and their mothers, the youngsters were set to work on puzzles. During intermission, mothers were told whether their offspring were doing well or poorly and were cautioned not to interfere. The investigators then left the room and watched from a hidden vantage point. They found that most firstborn immediately rushed to their mothers, who promptly praised those doing well and berated those doing poorly; later-born children did not turn to their mothers in this way.

Can prenatal influences affect health?

"The most significant period of an individual's life," an ancient Chinese philosopher observed, "is spent in his mother's womb." Modern research suggests he may have been right.

Among the most prized of medical X-ray films is one taken of the pelvis of a pregnant woman to determine whether or not she would be able to have a normal delivery. It showed, very clearly, the mouth of the fetus wide open, and the thumb inside the mouth, providing what some physicians consider to be some evidence that the emotional state of the mother may be reflected in the fetus.

It's easier, of course, to experiment with animals than with humans. Recent animal studies indicate that early experiences in the womb leave their marks. When, for example, researchers exposed pregnant rats to extreme crowding or loud noises, calculated to be upsetting to the mothers, their offsprings' teeth tended to chatter and the baby rats were slower than others in learning to run a maze. Moreover, the baby rats, when transferred to the care of foster mothers who had not been subjected to the same crowding or noises, remained abnormal. It seems likely that, since many substances pass from the maternal to the fetal bloodstream by means of the placenta, hormone changes and possibly other changes in mother rats may have affected their young. If this is so there could be some truth in the old wives' tales about prenatal influences and maternal impressions.

Some scientists point to the fact that the growth rate of the human brain reaches a peak at about the fifth month of fetal life, continues at this peak level until birth, then begins to level off. (The brain is already about 70 percent of its adult weight a few months after birth.) It seems logical to assume that both brain structure and brain functions can be influenced by conditions of life within the womb.

Actually, in animal studies, investigators have been able to demonstrate that hormones of the sexual, thyroid, and adrenal glands—which may be affected by stress upon the mother and may migrate across the placenta to the fetus—have a direct action on the nervous system of the young and if they act at a critical time in development, can produce permanent effects. For example, when the male hormone testosterone is injected into pregnant monkeys, the behavior of their female young is altered; although female in anatomy, they act like male offspring.

Recognizing that far too little as yet is known about prenatal influences, scientists are now intensifying research.

Is the birth process itself a factor in health?

All of us have a "touch of mental retardation or other blight" as a result of slight brain damage at birth, believes Dr. Abraham Towbin of Harvard Medical School. "Birth," he says, "is the most endangering experience to which most individuals are ever exposed."

Some measure of lack of oxygen and mechanical injury to the nervous system during birth seems to be inescapable. But until very recently, only the most obvious cases of birth damage were recognized. Severe lack of oxygen can produce mental retardation, cerebral palsy, or epilepsy. It is now known that mild lack of oxygen during birth may sometimes produce difficulties lumped together under the term "minimal brain dysfunction." Towbin estimates that minimal brain dysfunction may affect more than 3 million Americans, adults as well as children. They are characterized by behavioral disorders of varying degree, often accompanied by learning defects, reading difficulty, overactivity, or inordinate awkwardness.

If Towbin is right, minimal brain damage during birth may reduce a child's potential from the genius level to that of an average child or even less. It may spell the difference between two brothers, one a skilled athlete and the other an "awkward child." Much remains to be learned about slight brain damage in the newborn and how to prevent it.

Are environmental influences in early childhood
important to physical development?

It has been cocktail-party talk ever since Freud that emotional experiences in childhood can have lasting effects. Only recently, however, has there come to be any widespread awareness of the lasting physical effects of childhood influences.

The fact that contemporary Japanese teen-agers are now far taller than the typically short-statured Japanese of only a few decades ago obviously isn't the result of genetic change but of radical change in the Japanese way of life since World War II, including change in child-feeding and child-rearing patterns. Similarly, children born and raised on Israel's kibbutzim or collective settlements now often tower over parents who came from Central European ghettos.

Anywhere in the world that Western civilization's ways are adopted, children grow taller and faster and achieve sexual maturity earlier. Teen-age boys are much too big to fit into the armor of medieval knights; for girls, menstruation begins an average of three years earlier than it did a century ago.

Researchers have been able to demonstrate in laboratory experiments with animals the far-reaching and lasting effects of environmental influences early in life. Some of Dr. René Dubos' experiments at the Rockefeller University, New York, are particularly striking. When Dubos fed pregnant or lactating mice a diet somewhat smaller than usual or deficient in a vital substance such as magnesium, their offspring not only were unusually small at weaning but also stayed small for the rest of their lives even when, after weaning, they were fed everything they could possibly eat.

In another experiment, mice were mildly infected with a virus two days after birth. The mild infection produced no noticeable disease, but growth was depressed, and the growth inhibition persisted throughout the lives of the mice even though outwardly they appeared normal except for size.

Scientists are not yet sure why these physical influences have lifelong effect. One theory is that either nutritional deprivation or a minor infection could, if it occurred at a critical point in development, affect the hormone system, reducing the output of growth hormone, for example. Another theory is that nutritional deprivation early in life may lead to a lifelong reduction in the efficiency with which the body can utilize food.

In man and in animals, there appear to be critical periods for both physical and mental development, although they have not been clearly defined yet.

What early influences affect mental development?

Only thirty years ago, an authority on the subject described intelligence as an "inborn all-round intellectual ability, inherited or at least innate, not due to teaching and training." There are still some who argue that IQ is more a matter of inheritance than of environment and therefore can't be changed by education. And there are biologists who even today think in terms of being able to create a crop of Einsteins by making changes in genetic material, as though Einstein's experiences had nothing to do with his talent.

But the picture is hardly that simple. More and more researchers are convinced that while heredity plays a role, environment matters considerably. They talk in terms of environments rich and diversified in stimuli that favor nervous system and behavioral development, as measured by such things as exploratory activity, learning ability, and even chemical characteristics of the brain. They also talk of impoverished environments that may produce intellectual and behavioral deficiencies.

For normal development and functioning, sensory and social stimulation appear to be essential. In studies in which volunteers undertook to spend a few hours lying motionless in dark and soundless rooms, they soon began to suffer from hallucinations, twitching, and tics; hardly any wonder that solitary confinement has always been regarded as a severe kind of punishment.

Some years ago, Dr. Rene Spitz, a psychiatrist, studied two sets of infants. One set lived in a foundling home; the other lived in the nursery of a prison in which their mothers were inmates. In the foundling home cribs were separated from each other by partitions; in the prison there were no partitions. In the foundling home one nurse cared for seven or more babies; in the prison the babies were cared for by their delinquent mothers all day. Medical care was much the same in both institutions.

Yet Spitz found striking differences—even in resistance to disease. Over a three-year period there was no child death in the prison nursery, but more than one-third of the children in the foundling home died. All the prison babies learned to walk, talk, eat, and dress themselves at suitable ages; their heights and weights were normal. On the other hand, the foundling home children were retarded in every respect. Most did not learn such simple skills as walking, talking, and eating. And the retardation apparently was irreversible. When the foundling home babies reached sixteen months of age and were moved into a large sunny room free of partitions and with several nurses present throughout the day to care for and play with them, the children became progressively worse instead of better.

So tender loving care counts?

It may not be just a matter of TLC, though. When a baby is born, its mother instinctively cuddles, rocks, and makes sounds to it. From her standpoint, she is displaying love. She is also providing sensory stimulation. While love may be helpful, there is evidence from animal studies that stimulation is *essential*.

Experimenters have shown that stroking and handling newborn rats for only ten minutes a day helps them grow better. But they have obtained exactly the same results by tossing baby rats in the air, even by giving them mild electrical shocks. Rats so treated become larger, more active, less nervous, better able to learn, more resistant to infection. Some studies have demonstrated that infant rats handled only a few minutes a day, even roughly, grow up able to resist situations so stressful that they produce heart damage and ulcers in other adult rats.

As some behavioral scientists see it, a child's intelligence is fluid, ready to be expanded by contact with the environment. And they now know they can raise a child's IQ by as much as 25 points by means of environmental enrichment.

Has IQ actually been raised by environmental enrichment?

Yes. In a poor area of Milwaukee, Dr. Rick Heber of the University of Wisconsin found that of children with IQs under 80 (putting them in the retarded category) 80 percent had mothers with equally low IQs. This made it seem that the youngsters had inherited their lack of intelligence. But within three years after Heber set up a program of special training for newborn babies of such low-IQ mothers, the babies scored well above 100 in IQ.

In a Washington, D.C., ghetto Dr. Earl S. Schaefer—a developmental psychologist specializing in early childhood education—sent tutors into the homes of thirty children. For two years, an hour a day, five days a week, the tutors carried in puzzles, toys, and picture books, talked and played with the children, and took them on trips. At the end of two years, the thirty children, then three years old, had a mean IQ of 106. By contrast, a group of thirty similar children who were not helped had a mean IQ of 89, several were retarded, only three scored slightly above 100 in IQ. In the tutored group no child was retarded, and one had an IQ of 130.

The Schaefer study showed something else. When the thirty tutored children were four years old and out of the program for a year, their IQs began to drop. Other investigators report the same thing: first, large IQ changes with stimulation, then fall off when tutoring stops. What is needed is early and continuing stimulation.

With all the time, toys, and attention that middle-class parents lavish on their kids, why isn't IQ going up?

Actually, IQ generally seems to be on the rise. For example, World War II soldiers scored higher intellectually than World War I soldiers did. Half the men in World War II ranked as intelligent as the upper 5 percent of men in World War I.

After the Tennessee Valley Authority introduced new opportunities and stimulation into the lives of adults in what had been an isolated rural region, their children benefited. Among children reared after TVA, there was an average IQ gain of about 10 points compared with children reared pre-TVA.

"Wherever intellectual level has been followed, we're getting rises," says Dr. Joseph Hunt of the University of Illinois. He expects that intelligence may well continue to go up as culture becomes more complex and stimulating. "I am sure," he says, "that we have intellectual and linguistic skills far beyond what our ancestors had."

Are there any effects from separation of mother and child?

It's been almost taken for granted that disruption of a child's relationship with the most important individual in his environment, his mother, may have far-reaching effects. But just how severe the effects might be is a matter of dispute.

Since they can't perform many experiments on humans, investigators have resorted to animal studies, particularly with monkeys, hoping to use the results as models for understanding human behavior patterns.

At Cambridge University in England sixteen infant rhesus monkeys, aged twenty-one to thirty-two weeks, were separated from their mothers for a six-day period, two six-day periods, or a thirteen-day period. The infants were watched closely during separation and afterward when they were returned to their mothers.

As expected, when separated from its mother for a few days, an infant monkey calls a great deal at first, then shows a decrease in normal movement and play activity. More significantly, when studied six months and even two years later, the monkeys still showed much the same depressed motor and play activity that they did during the separation period. They tended to withdraw, shying away from strange objects and new experiences. Control monkeys, who had undergone no separation, showed no such symptoms. The British researchers think that separation effects may be somewhat similar for humans.

How important for adult health are childhood eating patterns?

Far more important than anyone has supposed until very recently. In Columbia, South America, a dark-haired little girl named Maria lives with her family in a shack on a steep hill overlooking the south side of the city of Bogota. She is four years old, yet she weighs only twenty-two pounds and is not yet three feet tall. Maria has an IQ of only 69; she is a victim of protein malnutrition.

At the Denver General Hospital in Colorado, nineteen children admitted between 1962 and 1967 at less than a year of age with generalized malnutrition scored poorly in intelligence when tested some years later.

These two examples suggest that dietary deficiencies in young children can retard intellectual development as well as physical well-being.

It is now clear that physical and mental apathy, long assumed to be racial or climatic in origin, is often the result of malnutrition. Investigators have found that populations deprived early in life often have little resistance to stress and escape disease only as long as little effort is required of them. They also find it difficult to execute long-range programs that could improve their status. They are, as René Dubos puts it, "prisoners of their nutritional past."

Among many recent studies, one in East Africa showed that Tanzanian children who received school snacks had better growth compared with control children who received no snacks. Also, the midday snacks reduced absenteeism and improved concentration, alertness, and learning. A study in Kentucky showed that children in schools where they received improved diets gained 30 months in mental age over a period of time. Children in other schools not providing improved diets gained only 15.5 months in the same period.

In several studies a small head circumference has been related to early malnutrition. Although there is little doubt that there is a close correlation between head circumference and brain size, there is no good exidence that brain size is related to intelligence. But investigators compared the brains of nine Chilean infants who had died of severe malnutrition with those of ten others who had died of accidents. They found a reduced number of brain cells in the malnourished children as compared with the others. It's not known how severe the malnutrition needs to be in order to reduce the number of brain cells nor what effects such reduction would have had on mental performance of these children had they survived.

René Dubos expresses his conviction in clear terms. "It can be unequivocally stated," he declares, "that the beneficial effects derived from building ultramodern hospitals with up-to-date equipment are trivial compared with the results that could be achieved with well-balanced food, sanitary conditions, and a stimulating environment."

Isn't the other extreme—overfeeding—harmful, too?

If obesity tends to shorten life—and there is evidence that it does—a common American pattern of feeding children may be a significant health-impairing, life-shortening factor: Give a child, day after day, too much food, and you can saddle him with a kind of physical sore spot.

The evidence comes from a whole series of recent studies. Dr. Jules Hirsch of Rockefeller University and Dr. Jerome Knittle of the Mount Sinai School of Medicine in New York City started with research in animals to see how early eating patterns affect later eating and growth. They used litters of rats broken up soon after birth and redistributed so that in some instances only four infant rats shared the milk of one mother while in other cases litters as large as twenty-two had to milk a single mother. At weaning, as might be expected, the rats from smaller litters were fatter, sleeker, and healthier looking than those from big litters.

After weaning, all the rats, lean and fat alike, were offered a diet with no quantity restrictions at all. It might be expected that the skinny, previously deprived rats would rush in and gobble large quantities and catch up with the others. Instead, the rats used to eating less went right on eating less; those used to eating more went on eating more. And while at first the fat rats beat out the skinny ones in growth, eventually the lean ones overtook them—and, in the end, the lean rats lived longer than the fat ones.

To find out why the eating habits of both groups did not change after weaning, Hirsch and Knittle carefully examined them at different ages. They found that at each age the fatter rats consistently had more fat cells than the skinny ones. And when the fat rats were put on restricted diets, their fat cells did not decrease in number, only in size. As soon as the diet restrictions were lifted, the fat cells shot up to previous size, and lost weight was promptly regained.

That may sound familiar to many persons who diet to lose

weight only to promptly regain the weight after the dieting. However, scientists have to be cautious about comparing rats and humans. To find out if the same thing might hold for humans, Knittle and an associate checked 200 children aged two to eighteen, all obese—i.e., at least 30 percent heavier than the ideal weight for their age. They removed a small sample of fat from each child and found that the number of fat cells in the tissue of these children was significantly greater than that in the tissue of youngsters of normal weight. In some instances, children only five or six years old had more fat cells than adults of normal weight.

Knittle went on to other studies showing that the fat cells of adults shrink and swell in direct relationship to food intake. He also found that the extra fat cells in obese adults seem to affect body metabolism in such a way that fat people must take in fewer calories to keep their weight down to ideal than people who had always remained at ideal weight.

A lean adult may have about 27 trillion fat cells in his body; an obese person, 77 trillion. And if, as it seems, all those extra fat cells keep sending out signals to be fed, they may help explain why food craving in the obese is not wholly psychological as some have thought but at least partly based on demand from an overpopulation of hungry fat cells.

The studies are especially important for parents. They provide insight into the need to establish good eating habits in children and thereby help them to avoid future difficulties.

There has long been a notion that a plump baby is a healthy one. It's been based on the supposition that a plump child is better equipped to stand disease. Quite commonly in the past fatness in babies was encouraged in order to help them withstand tuberculosis and other diseases. Even if the extra pounds ever did help, they certainly are not necessary now in view of modern medicine's ability to check such diseases.

*How do you tell the difference between a lean child
and an undernourished one?*

According to Dr. George Christakis, chief of the Nutrition Division at Mount Sinai School of Medicine, "There's a difference. The lean child is like the typical basketball player. His posture is good; his muscles are resilient; he's active and alert. The undernourished child has 'mushy' muscles, drooping shoulders, and a tendency to develop a pot belly, and he's tired and inactive a lot of the time."

Still, isn't it true that all children are not alike,
and obesity can stem from other factors?

It's true that children differ in tendencies to gain weight or
stay thin. And there may be an inherited predisposition one way
or the other. Some studies have shown that given two obese parents, a child has an 80 percent chance of being overweight. But
there is still a big question: Is the child's weight problem a
matter of inheritance or is it largely the result of eating habits
he learns from his parents?

It has also been found that patterns of activity distinguish
overweight children and those of normal weight. Dr. Jean Mayer
of Harvard, for example, found that obese high school girls he
studied didn't eat more but rather less than girls of normal
weight—and the girls in both groups were carefully matched for
height, social status, and intelligence—but the obese girls spent
two-thirds less time in exercise or physical activity of any kind.

Cornell researchers attached pedometers to infants' limbs to
record their activity. Their findings show that the relatively inactive babies become fat on the same amount of food on which
active babies stay at normal weight.

But while these factors do have an effect, and while there may
be emotional causes of overeating, the opinion of many investigators is expressed by Dr. Christakis: "It still seems that a major
basis of obesity is learned eating habits."

One recent report on the subject put it this way: "So apparently the real responsibility is placed upon parents, especially
mothers, who conciously or unconsciously form their children's
patterns of eating. Take, for example, a statement like, 'If you
don't clean your plate, you can't have any dessert.' This implies
that the child likes sweets better than meat or vegetables. And
why does he? Well—because mother does. So if women profit-
ably rethink their own attitudes toward food, they can pass on
healthy nutritional habits to their children."

Is it really true that most mothers want their kids to eat more?

A lot of interesting observations come from a recent study,
the most comprehensive nutritional study ever made of children
from birth to six years of age, as reported in *The New York
Times.*

It covered more than 3,000 preschool youngsters in 2,000
households in twelve states. The 2,000 families were white and
black, rich and poor, large and small, and lived in urban, sub-

urban, and rural areas. The great majority could afford good diets. An impressive 75 percent of mothers had attended nutrition classes; many reported learning about nutrition, too, from magazines, newspapers, and books.

Yet the study found a significant number of children overfed and undernourished, getting too many "empty" calories from candy, soft drinks, baked goods, and potato chips; too few from fruits and vegetables; and taking in too little vitamin A and vitamin C.

These were not careless mothers. They worried when their children weren't hungry at meal times (more than 75 percent), when they seemed to eat too little meat (20.5 percent), eat too little food (19.9 percent), drink too little milk (20.1 percent). To hear them tell it, their youngsters were "skin and bones." But they weren't. Many were obviously headed for a lifetime of overweight problems.

Few mothers worried that their children ate too much (2.9 percent). Many were concerned about sweets. Nearly 30 percent thought their four-year-olds ate too many sweets and drank too many soft drinks. Yet they might have solved the problem by keeping fewer sweets and soft drinks around the house and by not using sweets as rewards. Twenty-three percent of the mothers used food as a reward, and the most frequently given rewards were desserts and candy. These mothers had no idea that they were teaching their children to equate food with love, that they were setting up an emotional booby trap, and that in moments of stress later in life their offspring would turn to food for comfort and possibly stuff themselves to the point of obesity.

Do any other child-feeding practices have later consequences?

Starting a baby too soon on solid foods may head him toward a lifetime weight problem, according to Dr. S. L. Hammar and his research associates at the University of Washington. They recently compared overweight teen-agers with those of normal weight. Mothers of the obese adolescents reported that they had introduced solid foods at 6 weeks to 2 months; mothers of normal-weight counterparts reported introducing no solids until the third or fourth month. Hammar found a tendency among mothers to be competitive in advancing their babies by introducing new foods sooner than their neighbors. This sort of race, he found, is particularly common where mothers meet frequently to compare notes.

Dr. S. J. Fomon, professor of pediatrics at the University of

Iowa, suggests that too much intake of salt in infancy may predispose to high blood pressure later. Recently, he notes, manufacturers of baby foods have taken a healthy step by decreasing the salt content of a number of these foods.

Still another practice that needs scrutiny, Fomon thinks, is establishing a three-meals-a-day habit during early childhood. "Many parents appear to believe that the infant who eats three meals a day has achieved an important landmark in development. But animal studies provide rather convincing evidence that, at least in some species, consumption of small frequent feedings throughout the day is physiologically preferable to consumption of the same quantity of the same foods in one or two widely spaced meals. The meal-eating animals become obese, develop atherosclerosis, abnormal glucose tolerance, and heart disease. Thus, at least until more information is available on this point, urging infants and small children to adapt to a three-meals-a-day pattern seems unsound."

What's the answer?

Ideally, mothers should consult with pediatricians to work out a diet suited to the individual child's body build (see chapter 5), activity, and growth needs. Unhappily, not all pediatricians are competent to do this. In the past, half the medical schools in the country have offered inadequate nutrition education.

Hopefully, the time is coming when doctors will be more knowledgeable about diet, especially as research documents the importance of proper feeding and of the avoidance of overfeeding as well as undernutrition.

Are there unhealthy social attitudes about size?

About male height, yes. Cleveland sociologist Saul Feldman has observed that no matter what his race, creed, or financial status, an American male under 5 feet 8 inches is a victim of discrimination. So pervasive is the bias against the short man that no one except the short man even notices it. Take even the language. Instead of a neutral, "What is your height?" the question is always an invidious, "How tall are you?" A woman's idealized lover is never "short, dark, and handsome." The tall man, observes Feldman, has all of womankind to choose from while the short man must make do with the little woman.

Not only does the short man get short shrift in sports but business, too, apparently values height. Feldman points to a survey of recent University of Pittsburgh graduates, for instance, which shows that men 6 feet 2 inches and over received starting salaries averaging 12.4 percent higher than men under 6 feet tall. In another study, 140 corporate recruiters were asked to make a hypothetical choice between two equally qualified applicants, one 6 feet 1 inch and the other 5 feet 5 inches. Nearly 75 percent chose the tall man.

It's not what Feldman, who is 5 feet 4 inches tall, would call fair.

Does size affect health and longevity?

By and large, modern man stands a couple of inches taller and broader than the generation before him. If American kids are told they look big for their age, they can believe it. They're among the biggest in the world. A survey recently made by the National Center for Health Statistics found that American youngsters aged six through eleven have been growing steadily in height and weight for the last ninety years or more; they've gained about 10 percent in height on the average and their average weight has increased more than 15 percent.

Both black and white children have shared in the growth gain, with blacks tending to be slightly taller than whites, and the whites averaging slightly heavier.

Both boys and girls tend to gain height at a steady rate from six to twelve, although girls grow slightly faster than boys do during that age span. The boys, starting at an average height of 46.7 inches at six years of age, push up a bit more than 2 inches a year to 57.3 inches at age eleven. The girls grow about 2.3 inches a year, from 46.4 to 58.1. Weight gain also favors girls who go from being about half a pound less at age six to about 3.6 pounds heavier than boys at age eleven.

Our change in stature became apparent on a mass scale when the military in World War II had to tailor GI trousers as well as equipment to different dimensions than those they had used in World War I.

But if our burgeoning size has puffed up parental pride, it could, biologically, be a "false idol rather than ideal," suggests Dr. Richard S. Gubner, clinical professor of medicine at Downstate Medical Center in Brooklyn, New York.

During the Korean War, when autopsy studies were made on young American fatalities—youths who had only shortly before attained manhood—they showed that coronary atherosclerosis had developed in a large percentage, clogging the coronary arteries with fat deposits. This disease, long considered to be a degenerative one associated with age, was turning up in eighteen- and nineteen-year-olds. Wartime observations established that the youths of less affluent countries had neither the stature nor the coronary disease of American youth.

"The difference," says Dr. Gubner, "has been attributed to the fat-rich diet of American soldiers and, in general, much has been made of our high-fat diet compared with that of other nations. . . . But fat, sugar, and protein, and in general caloric abundance, as well as stress (also an American particularity) all stoke the same anabolic fire fanned by growth hormone. A reasonably good case may be made that this is the common metabolic pathway of affluence, affecting skeletal and adipose development and atherosclerosis."

Thus we are growing bigger at the expense of eating more and clogging our arteries—gaining stature at the cost of a longer, healthier life.

Is the increase in stature still going on?

There is some evidence that in well-nourished Americans it may have stopped.

One study of families in which four successive generations of sons went to Harvard University found that the oldest generation, born about 1858, produced sons on the average a little more than an inch taller than their fathers; but the fourth generation, born about 1941, showed no height increase.

Another study found that the height of boys entering Harvard from private schools in 1958–1959 had not increased over those of boys from such schools in the 1930s. That was also true of girls entering Wellesley from public or private schools. But the height of boys entering Harvard from public schools increased 1.5 inches during the period, which investigators believe is a result of improved living standards in lower socioeconomic groups.

Do we mature earlier?

Yes. Fifty years ago, maximum stature usually was not reached until age twenty-nine. Now, in affluent classes, it is commonly reached at nineteen in boys, seventeen in girls.

According to the eighteenth-century records of the Bach Boys Choir in Leipzig, Germany, the boys stopped singing soprano because of voice change at an average age of eighteen. A recent study of London schoolboys showed the average age of voice change to be 13.3 years.

Interestingly, too, the Bach Choir records show a sudden rise in the age of voice change during the 1740s when living standards in and around Leipzig fell because of the War of Austrian Succession. A similar phenomenon was noted in Moscow during World War II, when the average height of thirteen-year-old boys dropped by about an inch.

The age of onset of the menses, too, has been notably affected. On the average, it begins two to five years earlier than it did some years ago. In the seventeenth century, rural girls in Austria rarely reached menarche (began to menstruate) before their seventeenth, eighteenth, or even twentieth year. In 1820 working-class girls in Manchester, England, reached menarche on the average at 15.7 years. In 1934 a study of New York girls showed an average age of 13.53 years at menarche. The most recent studies, including one of more than 6,000 student nurses, show menses appearing midway between twelve and thirteen years.

Some investigators believe that a new trend is developing. The drop in the age of menarche appears to be leveling off in the more affluent populations. According to Dr. Alan E. Treloar of the National Institute of Child Health and Human Development, who recently has been studying 1,500 Minnesota women and their daughters, it may even have reversed. Within the last decade the average age of menarche in this group has risen slightly. This could mean either that some factor other than nutrition is at work, which is contrary to general belief, or that the traditional value of some American diets has deteriorated.

A study of Dr. Isabelle Valadian at Harvard suggests that the diet of soft drinks and candy bars favored by some girls before puberty has an effect on the reproductive tract, leading to poor childbearing histories later. Dr. Valadian has followed up on girls whose nutritional histories had been recorded earlier by Dr. Harold C. Stuart at Harvard. Those girls marked low on childhood diet had a significantly greater number of unsuccessful pregnancies than those ranked high in nutrition.

Is there anything other than nutrition that could account for earlier maturity?

Other possible factors have been explored. The idea that earlier menarche occurs in hot, humid climates, for example, has been discredited.

As for racial differences, the mean age of menarche for girls in Nigeria is 14.22 years; for Alaskan Eskimo girls, it is 14.42 years. Chinese girls in Hong Kong and Cuban girls of predominantly Negro stock experience menarche at about the same time as Eurpoean girls. If the Cuban and Chinese girls were better fed, some investigators believe, they might possibly mature even earlier. But racial differences seem to have slight influence in comparison with varying living standards.

Nor do psychological influences, such as early association with boys, seem significant. Girls in co-ed schools do not reach menarche any sooner than those in girls' schools.

But there is an interesting hypothesis suggested recently by Dr. Rose E. Frisch and Dr. Roger Revelle of the Harvard Center for Population Studies. They believe that menarche is initiated when the body reaches a critical weight. Just before puberty there is a growth spurt. It begins when weight, averaged for any age group, reaches about 68 pounds. Menarche itself occurs at a mean weight of 106 pounds. And it seems to occur without regard to age or height. It could explain why earlier rapid body growth has led to earlier puberty.

One study that helps buttress the hypothesis found an altitude effect—a delaying effect—on menarche. The effect was noted when comparisons were made of figures for growth and date of menarche obtained by the Child Research Center in Denver (5,300 feet altitude) and those obtained by the Guidance Council in Beverly Hills, California (sea level). In both cases, the girls were upper middle class and well nourished. The Denver girls averaged 7 pounds at birth and their mean age at menarche was 13.1 years. The California girls averaged 7.5 pounds at birth and reached menarche at a mean age of 12.8 years. The lower birth weight and the slower growth rate of the Denver girls—they lagged behind the California girls in weight gain throughout development—were attributed to the relative oxygen shortage at high altitude. But when they finally reached menarche, their average weight was much the same as it was for the California girls upon reaching menarche.

If people mature earlier, will they age earlier and have shorter life-spans?

In recent years, the earlier increase in life-span associated with medical advances has leveled off, despite continuing medical advances. Some investigators believe there is a possibility that this could be the result of earlier maturation.

But they also admit that such an effect would not be easy to pinpoint. They note, too, that menopause in women is occurring somewhat later than before, indicating an opposite effect. As far back as the fourth century B.C., Aristotle wrote: "The menses

cease in most women around the fortieth year." Today, menopause tends to occur at about fifty; but trends are not easy to
establish clearly because of widespread use of hormone pills
both for birth control and to ease the effects of menopause.

Do children of divorce have special problems?

Millions of emotional words have been written about divorce,
which now ends one in every four marriages in the United States.
But there has been little solid fact. And there still is no definitive
information about any effects of divorce on the physical health
and longevity of children.

But one long-term study sheds some light on other aspects. It
indicates that children of divorce never emerge completely un-
scathed. The study by Dr. Judson T. Landis of the University of
California at Berkeley used data obtained over a thirteen-year
period from 3,000 male and female college students at the
University of California and eleven other institutions across the
country. Landis found that boys and girls from divorced families
generally start dating later. They date fewer persons and date
less frequently than teen-agers from happy homes who often date
as many as twenty members of the opposite sex before marriage.
But kids from broken homes go steady more often and have more
private understandings about engagements, apparently because
they seek security.

Children of divorced parents often report feeling different
from others, inferior, or ashamed of the divorce; they have less
confidence in their ability to establish normal relations with the
opposite sex; a larger percentage of them want to be of the
opposite sex than do adolescents from happy families. However,
children of divorce boast higher marks in school, suggesting that
by working for grades they may attempt to compensate for feelings of inadequacy.

Emotional shock of a child during divorce of his parents is
closely linked to how the child judges his home before the divorce. Shock is greatest among those who have believed their
parents to be happy, as three out of four do. They have difficulty
adjusting to the sudden discovery. For these children, even death
is easier to understand than divorce. They feel that if a mother
could reject a father, she could reject a child, too. On the other
hand, children not surprised by divorce find relief when it actually comes; they have more security and happiness afterward
because there is less tension in their lives.

Does continued home conflict hurt children more than divorce?

Such marriages, Dr. Landis' study indicated, tend to be more disturbing to a child than the fact of divorce. "It isn't the divorce but the unhappy home situation that determines how a child will meet life as he grows up," says Dr. Landis.

There's an interesting study on unstable childhood and the mental problems of physicians. Like anyone else, physicians can have psychiatric problems. In fact, they may have more than their share of them.

Twice as many doctors as nondoctors showed at least two of three conditions frequently looked upon as occupational hazards of medical practice—bad marriage, psychiatric problems for which treatment is sought, and relatively heavy drug use—according to a thirty-year follow-up study reported by Dr. George E. Vaillant of Tufts University School of Medicine in Boston. But the study indicated that an unstable childhood, rather than the work of medicine, is the primary cause of such problems among physicians.

The study began thirty years ago, when forty-seven college sophomores who later went to medical school and seventy-nine other sophomores who later went into other fields were selected. None had any easily detectable mental or physical health problems, and all easily met academic standards. Over the thirty years, all were followed by questionnaires and occasional interviews.

There were no differences between the doctors and the others in terms of socioeconomic status on college entrance and no difference in intellectual aptitude. When they reached midlife, the doctors on the average made more money ($35,000–$40,000) than the others. Yet almost half the doctors had bad marriages, a third sought relief from drugs, and a third had undergone psychotherapy. The doctors required hospitalization at some time during the thirty years for alcoholism, depression, or functional physical complaints at a rate three times higher than the rate for nondoctors.

Such a disparity cannot be explained simply by stresses encountered by doctors as part of their work. While such stresses may be partially responsible for alcoholism and drug addiction, and while the medical sophistication of physicians may lead to greater uses of psychiatry, the study pointed to unstable childhood as responsible for the most part.

The physician group, Dr. Vaillant notes, included more per-

sons who had had unstable or unsupportive childhoods. Looking at the nondoctors and doctors as a group, only one in seven
of the men with the most supportive childhoods experienced
psychiatric problems, whereas almost half the men with relatively unstable childhoods had such symptoms.

A major factor in an unstable childhood, the study found,
was the "distant" parent. And it appears that "the long hours,
the demanding patients, the fact he is home late for supper, the
ready access to narcotics, are no problems to the doctor whose
childhood has been happy."

Is it true that family structure in general is breaking down?

Today's families are in deep trouble, and the reasons lie not
so much in the family itself as in the institutions of society,
according to Professor Urie Bronfenbrenner of the Cornell
University Department of Human Development and Family
Studies. There is today what he calls "pollution of the social environment." He sees an emergence of a pattern of life that puts
children and families last.

Society is imposing pressures and priorities, says Bronfenbrenner, that allow neither time nor place for meaningful activities and relationships between children and adults. Society expects its citizens, first of all, to meet job demands and fulfill civic
and social obligations; responsibilities to children are to be met,
but for many this is spare-time activity. The frustrations are
greatest for the poverty-stricken family but there's a rat race
even for families with more money.

As factors that help to isolate children from the rest of society
Bronfenbrenner cites the fragmentation of the extended family,
the separation of residential and business areas, the disappear-
ance of the neighborhoods, and occupational mobility. He also
includes television, separate patterns of social life for different
age groups, the working mother, and the delegation of child care
to specialists. The primary danger of TV, he believes, lies not so
much in the behavior it produces as in the behavior it prevents—
the talks, games, family festivities, and arguments that contribute to a child's learning and character formation.

What is needed, he thinks, is a change in the family patterns
of living to bring people back into the lives of their children and
children back into the lives of people. Short of this change, there
will be even more rapid growth of alienation, apathy, drugs,
delinquency, and violence among the young, the not-so-young,

and all segments of national life. He feels it is essential to work to develop institutions and attitudes that will encourage a re-arrangement of both social and business life in order to make possible more meaningful interaction of adults with children.

5

Body Build, Body Rhythms, Intelligence, and Education

Does one's body type have any effect on how long one will live?

People have been intrigued for centuries by the relationship between body types and disease and longevity—and by any possible relationship between body types and emotional structure and behavoir. Only recently, however, has there been serious scientific study. And there is evidence that each person may have more or less proneness—or, conversely, more or less resistance—to a number of important problems according to his body type.

What are the types?

Although no two human bodies are exactly alike—in fact, the ways in which they differ are virtually endless—in certain aspects there are degrees of likeness among large groups.

As far back as Hippocrates, around 450 B.C., two basic body types were recognized. One, the phthisic, was long and thin and was considered to be particularly susceptible to tuberculosis and respiratory diseases. The other, the apoplectic, was short and thick and was considered to be prone to stroke (apoplexy).

These types were pretty broad. And it wasn't until the 1700s that a four-type system was proposed: abdominal type, muscular type, respiratory type, and cerebral type. Each was believed to be more susceptible to some diseases than to others. More recently, three basic constitutional types were suggested: pyknic, or sthenic (short, fat, heavy); athletic (muscular, broad, strong); and asthenic (thin, weak, slender).

An American physician, W. H. Sheldon, in the 1930s established the modern classification: endomorphs, mesomorphs, and ectomorphs.

Sheldon sorted out photographs of 4,000 American college students of many races and ethnic groups and found three extremes of body shape. The extreme endomorph is rounded, has a round head, a bulbous stomach, a heavy build, a lot of fat, yet is not necessarily a fat person. The mesomorph, in the extreme, has a large head, broad shoulders, a lot of bone and muscle, not much fat, and relatively narrow hips. The ectomorph is thin, all angles and sharpness, with spindly arms and legs, narrow shoulders, still narrower hips, and not much fat or muscle.

Sheldom was able to show that in any large group of men or boys chosen at random, the three basic body types would be present. He also established that any one person is not entirely one type; rather, he shows varying degrees of each, though one type usually predominates.

Sheldon devised a method for grading the various overlapping characteristics found in individual body builds (somatotypes), and he developed a scientific terminology for these somatotypes that could be used descriptively and would have the same meaning for investigators everywhere. He judged the amount of each characteristic possessed by each of his 4,000 pictured males and rated these amounts from 1 to 7. The smallest degree of a single characteristic an individual might have is designated as 1, the most as 7.

The three extremes, the very round endomorph, the Hercules-like mesomorph, and the very thin ectomorph, were classified as 7-1-1, 1-7-1, and 1-1-7, respectively. A man with equal amounts of all three characteristics was rated 4-4-4. One with some of the shoulder features of a mesomorph and some of the roundness of an endomorph but with much more of the narrow angularity of an ectomorph might be classified as 3-3-5 or 2-2-6.

The system is not simple but aided by use of standard photographs different investigators do, in fact, arrive at nearly identical classifications. Actually, Sheldon refined the system into many minor classifications until finally he had seventy-six different somatotypes. But these classifications usually have meaning only for specialists.

Can one determine one's own somatotype?

To a degree. If you examine your naked body in a mirror, you may arrive at no precise scientific evaluation but you'll come reasonably close.

Characteristic endomorphic features include roundness and softness of body, predominance of abdomen; high, square shoulders; short neck; large head; wide face; short limbs; small bones; and soft, smooth skin much like that of an apple. There is often a premature tendency to baldness. It's possible to be an endomorph without being obese, but the extreme endomorph most often does become obese.

Mesomorphic features include squareness and hardness of body; rugged muscling; large prominent bones; large trunk; bigger chest than abdomen; fairly long neck; low waist; thick and relatively coarse skin, often with large pores; long, broad face; and somewhat coarse hair, which may be either luxuriant or sparse.

Ectomorphic features include linearity and delicacy, almost fragility of body; small bones; slight muscles; drooping shoulders; relatively short trunk with long limbs (though not necessarily tall); flat abdomen; narrow rounded shoulders which are often carried well forward so the arms may seem to hang in front of the body; relatively long arms; long and slender neck; slight head; delicate, thin lips; thin, dry skin; and fast-growing, fine hair.

How does somatotype relate to personality?

According to Sheldon's findings, the extreme endomorph tends to be a "comfortable" person fond of soft bed and soft furniture, and virtually all comforts. He does well socially, is interested in the problems of others and has tolerance for their faults. He expresses his feelings readily. And he loves food; it is one of the great interests of his life.

The extreme mesomorph is seemingly full of energy, and loves physical activity and competition. He behaves aggressively, walks and talks assertively, stands and sits upright. His concerns tend to be with the present rather than with the past or future. Where the extreme endomorph is one kind of extravert (of affect), the extreme mesomorph is another kind (of action).

The extreme ectomorph is introverted, doesn't fit in well in crowds, and tends to be an outsider, and an observer rather than participator. He is interested in ideas. When he faces problems, he often seeks solitude to solve them. He is sensitive to noise and distractions and tends to have many functional complaints such as insomnia, chronic fatigue, and allergies.

Just as there is overlapping of body build features, there is overlapping of personality traits.

How does somatotype relate to disease?

Even before Sheldon's classification was published, the great physician, Sir William Osler, was aware that among his patients with coronary heart disease there were no ectomorphs. In 1928 Dr. Samuel Levine, a distinguished heart specialist, specifically observed that most of his heart patients had round forearms rather than the flat ones characteristic of ectomorphs. A study of young coronary patients found that the majority were mesomorphs. Later, another study involving autopsies of thirty-eight men who had died from coronary heart disease showed that 63 percent had been mesomorphs and only 8 percent were ectomorphs.

From these studies, it appears that more often than not a coronary heart patient, particularly the middle-aged or younger patient, has a mesomorphic constitution.

Says Dr. Meyer Friedman, a well-known heart researcher of San Francisco: "Perhaps the fairest manner of presenting our opinion about the relationship of mesomorphy to coronary artery disease is to state the fact that when we first see and examine a tall, quite thin, poorly muscled individual with flat forearms who is less than fifty-five years of age, we would be rather surprised if he were found to have clinical coronary artery disease."

Dr. Menard M. Gertler of New York University has reported that when a group of young coronary heart attack patients is compared with a similar group of young individuals who have not suffered the disease, the coronary group consists of 25.7 percent endomorphs as against 29.9 percent in the control group; 42.2 percent mesomorphs in the coronary group, 19.8 percent in the control group; and 7.3 percent ectomorphs in the coronary and 21.1 percent in the control group.

In Gertler's study not only do mesomorphs in the coronary group outnumber those in the control group by more than 2 to 1; an overwhelming number of the endomorphs and ectomorphs in the coronary group show strong mesomorphy as the second dominant feature. It appears that one's body build is related to degree of proneness to coronary heart disease, with mesomorphs and endormorphic mesomorphs most vulnerable, ectomorphs least vulnerable.

In the government's Framingham study 198 men who developed coronary heart disease within twelve years of entry into the study were significantly more endomorphic and less ectomorphic than the 1,427 men who did not. The Framingham study found that physique contributed to the risk of coronary heart disease independently of blood pressure and serum cholesterol. If blood pressure and cholesterol were normal, physique alone could triple the relative risk. If pressure and cholesterol were elevated too, on top of a 3-to-1 increased physique risk, the total risk went up still higher.

Sheldon found that victims of gallbladder disorders—about four-fifths of whom are women—are usually mesomorphic endomorphs.

Cancer is a disease of many varieties and there has not yet been enough study of the role of physique in relation to cancer. But Sheldon found that there apparently is a remarkable degree of immunity to all forms of cancer among mesomorphic ectomorphs and that cancer appears to be rare in all pronounced ectomorphs.

Do endomorphs tend to become obese?

Body build does seem to be related to obesity. In a study of obese adolescent girls, Dr. Carl C. Seltzer and Dr. Jean Mayer of Harvard found them to be clearly more endomorphic, somewhat more mesomorphic, and considerably less ectomorphic than nonobese girls of comparable age.

Dr. Mayer states: "Presumably, then, the prime prerequisite for the development of obesity is a physique with at least a moderate amount of endomorphy under normal nutritional conditions. Endomorphy, which is neither a disease nor a sin, is an inherited predisposition to the laying on of fat unless insufficient diet, great activity, disease, or voluntary weight control supervenes."

It is not known if these findings apply to adults. Being a scientist, Dr. Mayer cautions that until further studies are done, the findings for obese adolescent girls should be applied to obese men and women only with some reserve. "In adults particularly, the problem of obesity is much more complex, because among them are physical types which are prone in middle age to a sudden blossoming into obesity. Any study of adults, therefore, must distinguish between those whose obesity is long-standing, going back to childhood and adolescence, and those for whom it is a singular characteristic of mid-life. Actually, our preliminary studies in adult women suggest that in middle age, as in adolescence, not all physical types are equally prone to become obese. There, too, very ectomorphic types with long, narrow hands and feet just do not become obese."

Would it be true to say that body type can dictate obesity?

No. All scientists emphasize that while body type may predispose one toward obesity, it is not the direct cause of obesity. So although the tendency is there, individual endomorphs have individual differences in the tendency. Some stay thin.

Ectomorphy, on the other hand, seems to confer a special ability to avoid the accumulation of fat. "Nature," Dr. Mayer observes, "seems to be intolerant of obesity in ectomorphic types. People so blessed may apparently follow the dictates of their appetite without fear of growing fat."

An endomorph or a mesomorph who gains weight while eating no more than an ectomorph—and that's a familiar phenomenon —can blame his body type, but only for making it necessary to eat a little less or expend more calories in physical activity than the ectomorph.

Even if body build does predispose, Dr. Mayer says, "This in no way detracts from the concept that caloric intake in excess of caloric expenditure is the immediate cause of obesity."

Do food needs differ according to body type?

Sheldon himself believed that it was necessary to learn how to feed the different somatotypes, that here was a real chance to test the old adage "One man's meat is another man's poison."

"We have picked up a number of preliminary clues," he reported. "It is clear that the ectomorph needs to eat oftener than the endomorph or mesomorph and that the mesomorphic ectomorph requires more food per unit of body weight than is needed by other somatotypes. These mesomorphic ectomorphs seem especially to need protein in large quantity. This may be true even in the later decades of life."

He also observed, "When endomorphy predominates there is usually a fairly strong craving for sweets. Does this represent a biological need of some sort? Should carbohydrates be limited when endomorphy is high or should these people follow their own inner impulses?"

Sheldon noted that the endomorph has a larger, heavier intestine than the ectomorph and wondered whether that meant that there ought to be two quite different diets for endomorphs and ectomorphs.

He was in favor of systematic research that might provide a rational plan for optimum feeding of the different somatotypes with some hope that such feeding might help to increase disease immunity and resistance to infection. Such research remains to be completed.

Is there any connection between intelligence and longevity?

There's some evidence that there may be a relationship. According to current studies by Dr. Eric Pfeiffer of Duke University, no one factor determines longevity, but a constellation of biologic, psychologic, and social factors provides a kind of "elite status." People with high intelligence, sound financial status, well-maintained health, and intact marriages may expect to live longer than their less intelligent and poorer brothers and sisters whose health is declining and whose marriages are no longer intact.

In the studies, long-term survivors have mean intelligence-test scores significantly greater than the short-term survivors, and the mean number of years of education is greater for the long-term survivors.

But can intelligence be measured clearly enough?

No, and that's part of the problem of assessing its influence. Although the intelligence quotient concept is one of the oldest and most thoroughly studied in psychology, it escapes precise definition.

Many people who have taken intelligence tests, especially if they failed to do as well as they thought they should, have been convinced that an IQ score doesn't tell the whole story about intelligence. Many psychologists agree. Traditional intelligence tests don't fully indicate intellectual status, although they have some usefulness. They were devised more than sixty years ago to determine which children could not learn at normal rates. And they emphasize abilities bearing on school learning in such key subjects as reading and arithmetic. They seem to predict less well beyond elementary grades, as subjects become more varied. And even at elementary levels, when it comes to early learning in reading and spelling, their predictions leave much to be desired.

How do IQ tests work?

An IQ is derived by presenting a student with a variety of standard questions. Based on how many he answers correctly, he is assigned a "mental age." The mental age is divided by the student's actual chronological age to determine his IQ. For example, an eight-year-old who has a mental age of ten would have an IQ of 1.25. By custom, the decimal point is shifted two places to the right and the IQ is expressed as 125. An IQ of 100 is average.

Traditional IQ tests have been under attack and, in fact, public schools in some large metropolitan areas have abandoned them on the grounds that the scores for ghetto children are misleading, sometimes classifying really bright students as dull and spoiling their futures when the truth may be that their poor scores are simply the result of an inadequate command of English.

IQ tests, some critics say, really don't assess intelligence at all but rather test what a student has learned. The test results commonly help determine whether children are put into "slow" or "fast" classes, which career programs they eventually enter, and, many critics say, what teachers expect of them. This last is believed by some educators to be a crucial element in student performance. Teacher expectation, they say, tends to become a self-fulfilling prophecy.

Are there any other tests?

Several other intelligence tests are based on the concept that it's possible to tell how smart an individual is by presenting him with stimuli—flashing a light in the eyes, for example. The light produces tiny changes in brain waves and the changes may reflect intelligence. The quicker the changes, the smarter the individual; the slower, the duller.

The instrument for this purpose, called a "neural efficiency analyzer," has produced some interesting results in early studies. It was invented by Dr. John Ertl, a University of Ottawa psychologist, who himself had scored only 77 on a conventional IQ test but later was able to establish that his IQ was actually 140.

To take a test with the neural efficiency analyzer, a subject dons a helmet containing electrodes that rest lightly atop his head. He looks at a light that flashes about once a second for two minutes. The electrodes pick up brain waves, which are then amplified and fed to a computer for analysis.

In some 6,500 subjects studied in this way, the speed of brain-wave response correlated well, but not exactly, with standard IQ scores. The exceptions appear to be important. For example, in a study with 1,000 Canadian schoolchildren, the analyzer gave relatively high scores to seven youngsters who, on the basis of IQ tests, had been assigned to "slow" classes. The seven were put into regular classes, where they proceeded to do successful work.

Nobody knows what the instrument really measures, but it probably doesn't measure intelligence in itself, which, says Dr. Ertl, "is a concept equivalent to truth and beauty. I don't know what intelligence is, but I do know what it is not. It's not the score on an IQ test, and it is not what our equipment measures." But he insists that his measurement is more valid than IQ tests in terms of assessing the brain's biological efficiency. He draws this conclusion because the measurement completely avoids cultural influences, requires no language, and involves no conscious response.

The neural efficiency analyzer is just one of the ways investigators are beginning to probe the mind by studying how the brain reacts to changes in the world around it, changes ranging from flashing lights and beeping sounds to shocks and even puffs of air. Some believe such research may open the way to the first intelligence and personnel tests that are fair to minority cultures and races.

Is IQ established at birth?

The idea that it is an immutable, God-bestowed ability, a constant fixed at birth, is dead. There is increasing evidence that IQ fluctuates substantially throughout early life.

Many studies, for example, show a depressive effect of environment on IQ scores. Among them are findings of a distinct rise in mean scores in populations over a period of time when changes occur that cut unemployment rates, improve nutrition, and broaden educational opportunities. IQ gains have been noted in young children from institutions for the retarded as well as from slum families after the children were given special teaching.

Some research suggests that a critical period for the development of IQ in many children may be between twelve months and thirty months. Unless there is organic brain damage or a genetic condition such as mongolism—and the incidence of both is relatively small—it is this eighteen-month period that may largely determine a child's intellectual level for life.

The implications in the mental retardation area are great. As many as 4.5 million of the 6 million Americans now considered mentally retarded may not be retarded at all in the classic sense. They are victims of misfortune, of social and cultural deprivation, who were given no chance in the critical eighteen-month period to perform as well as others. Their condition, then, may be preventable; for many it may still be reversible.

What's the evidence that environment affects IQ?

Two recent studies revealed little if any difference between minority and white students in intelligence and achievement test scores when social and environmental factors were considered. And the studies are believed to present the strongest evidence yet in documenting that environmental and social factors influence test scores.

When she found a disproportionate number of black and Chicano children in classes for the mentally retarded in Riverside, California, Dr. Jane Mercer of the University of California looked for possible causes. She discovered that the black and Chicano students whose families were like those of average middle-class whites had IQs equal to the whites. Also, the IQ tests used were as much as 30 percent based on cultural background. When this background was accounted for, Dr. Mercer found, the average IQ for all three groups was essentially the same.

Her study was a local one. But Dr. George W. Mayeske of the U.S. Office of Education made a nationwide analysis. He found that achievement test scores of minority and white children were almost identical when environmental and social factors were cancelled out statistically.

Some of the socioeconomic factors involved in both studies were the amount of space in homes, presence of mothers who expected children to go beyond high school, fathers with more than nine years of schooling, families speaking English all or most of the time, families owning their own homes.

Is intelligence linked to physical fitness?

Certainly, physical fitness doesn't guarantee superior mental achievement, but there's overwhelming evidence that it's related to general learning potential.

The eminent cardiologist, Dr. Paul Dudley White, titled one of his reports "The Brain, Too, Has Arteries." In it, he declared that the development and maintenance of intellectual health depended in large part upon good circulation to the brain. Such circulation depended upon the blood-pumping capacity of the leg muscles and the action of the diaphragm. And exercise, especially involving the legs, was mandatory to improve and maintain adequate blood supply to the brain.

White's contention has been supported by investigators who used instruments to check on heartbeat, breathing, blood pressure, and other physical factors. They demonstrated that during mental tasks there are changes in such factors, indicating that mental work is dependent on mobilization of energy and the condition of the circulatory system, as well as nervous system.

And there have been studies upsetting old misconceptions about gifted children. After twenty-five years of examining brilliant children, Lewis M. Terman, a Stanford University psychologist, concluded, "The results of the physical measurements and medical examinations provide a striking contrast to the popular stereotype of the child prodigy, so commonly predicted as a pathetic creature, over-serious, undersized, sickly, hollow-chested, nervously tense, and bespectacled, but the truth is that almost every element in the picture, except the last, is less characteristic of the gifted child than of the mentally average."

Supporting Terman's findings are other studies showing that gifted children not only have a high degree of academic superiority but they also, both girls and boys, are superior in height, weight, and grip strength. Still other studies have found that where only 2.35 percent of students above average in scholarship are below average in physique, 39.7 percent of those with poor scholarship are below average in physique.

Recently, after viewing all the latest evidence, the President's Council on Physical Fitness observed, "It may be contended that a person's general learning potential for a given level of intelligence is increased or decreased in accordance with his degree of physical fitness."

*Does current brain research hold any implications
for health and longevity?*

Decidedly yes. The complexity of the human brain has always staggered the imagination. A 3.5-pound mass, small enough to be held in the palm of the hand, it contains 10 billion cells, each of which may have 60,000 junction points. It uses no more power than a flashlight. How does it think, remember, create, adapt to change, guide the body to survival?

Researchers are beginning to get answers—and in the process they are uncovering findings of import for health. Using sophisticated instruments and techniques, they have mapped the brain and nervous system, traced major circuits, and have begun to relate the circuits and components to behavior.

There now begins to be some promise of brain prostheses, or appliances, for the blind and deaf and for victims of stroke, spinal cord injury, and other crippling diseases. As analysis of brain structure progresses, there is increasing likelihood of finding the causes of mysterious diseases such as multiple sclerosis.

Epilepsy control has already been achieved in about 75 percent of patients treated with anticonvulsant drugs; but new and more effective drugs are badly needed for the others. They may well come from brain studies. Witness the story of L-dopa, a new drug treatment for Parkinson's disease. It came as the result of brain-study techniques allowing determinations of how individual brain cells can be made defective through deficiencies of certain chemicals.

Some of the brain studies begin to suggest the possibility of ultimate chemical control over memory, learning speed, and, some scientists think, even intelligence.

Does education have any significant effect on health and longevity?

Greater income, satisfaction with job, and happier marriage, for example, apparently contribute to health and longevity (we'll discuss these factors later). So it can be assumed that education may be of considerable influence.

A study sponsored by the Carnegie Commission on Higher Education and reported in 1971 indicates that people who have gone to college tend to be more satisfied with their jobs, more highly paid, less subject to unemployment, and happier in marriage.

When it comes to income, the median for a family head with only a grammar school education was $5,170; for one with some high school education, $7,260; for a high school graduate, $8,940; for a person with some college education but no degree, $9,610; for a college graduate, $11,240; for one with advanced college or professional education or degree, $13,120.

As for job satisfaction, 89 percent of those with college degrees found their work enjoyable, as against 78 percent of those with high school educations, and still fewer with less education. More than three times as many of the least educated as compared with the more educated found their work sheer drudgery.

Where only 38 percent of those with grade school and 46 percent of those with high school educations evaluated their marriages as being very happy, 60 percent of college graduates did. An additional 22 percent of college graduates classified their marital happiness as above average compared with 16 percent of the least educated.

The Carnegie study report notes that there are exaggerated notions about the dollar value of higher education. The main point, according to the report, is more subtle. College-educated people hold jobs that expose them to fewer accidents and income losses, that offer more advancement, and that depend less on physical capacity and are more sympathetic to the aging process.

What about body rhythms—the internal clocks— and longevity?

This is a vast new area with tremendous implications for health and longevity. It's beginning to give the old question, "What makes a person tick?" new significance.

Body rhythms are biological ups and downs, apparently under the control of built-in body clocks. The best-known example is the way body temperature varies with time of day, being a little lower in the morning than in the evening in most people. But there are many other rhythms, including daily cycles in heartbeat rate, the number of white corpuscles circulating in the blood, adrenal hormone secretions, brain-wave activity, blood pressure, excretion of urinary substances, even the division of cells that make up organs and tissues.

Does everybody have these rhythms?

They are present not only in all people but in all living things. One demonstration of internal clocks in animals is the way a dormouse arouses itself from winter hibernation every three weeks or so and always at a time near sunset. You see a plant's clock in operation when its petals open before dawn even when you exclude all indications of sunrise.

One demonstration of man's biological clocks is the dulling of mental acuity in travelers who jet across a succession of time zones. Studies made by scientists for the Federal Aviation Agency show clearly that it's the inability of the body to readjust its rhythms quickly that generates both mental and physical fatigue.

To prove that the fatigue reactions don't come from just the duration of flight time, scientists tested three teams of travelers, consisting of four men each, who were flown from Oklahoma City to Rome (fourteen hours) and Manila (twenty-six hours) and from Washington, D.C., to Santiago, Chile (eighteen hours). In the men who crossed many time zones (six to Rome, ten to Manila) the investigators found significant changes in physical and psychological functioning. But in the men crossing only one time zone on the largely north-south flight to Santiago, there was virtually no change.

When, for example, it was 5:00 P.M. in Rome, the men's bodies, still synchronized to United States time, functioned as if it were 11:00 P.M. Their breathing and heart rates had dropped, and body temperatures were down as they would normally be late at night. The men had slept on the plane but they still felt tired. And, when tested, they showed marked impairment in their ability to concentrate or make decisions. They needed as much as 30 percent more time than usual for example, to add a row of two-digit numbers. Most of the psychological disturbances were gone within twenty-four hours, but many physical disruptions lasted three to five days.

As a result of such studies, many physicians in industry now advise a day of rest for executives after long east- or west-bound flights to important business conferences.

Do rhythms vary from person to person?

They do, which helps to explain why some of us are morning people who get up bright and cheerful in the morning, full of energy, while others are night owls who get up surly and may need several cups of coffee before they can get started. But later in the day the night owls are at their best while the morning people become less vigorous.

Ideally, individual work schedules should be synchronized with individual body rhythms. At least some people—mostly those in the creative arts—can and do match their body rhythms and their work hours. Many writers, for example, believe they do their best work late in the day. Ernest Hemingway, on the other hand, was an early bird who started writing very early in the morning and continued to noon.

Do rhythms affect one's performance?

Any attempt to completely defy body clocks can produce significant efficiency impairment. Studies by the U.S. Air Force's Aerospace Medical School have shown that when pilots were forced to work against their body rhythms, their performance fell by as much as 50 percent.

By and large, tasks demanding skill are performed more efficiently during the daytime, the hours when hormone levels are relatively high; and the best time for social activity is in the evening, when hormone levels are relatively low. Some recent studies at the Institute for Flight Medicine, in Bad Godesberg, West Germany, show that peaks of mental performance and physical fitness generally occur between 1:00 P.M. and 7:00 P.M. when most body cycles are in their active phase, while poorest response occurs between 2:00 A.M. and 6:00 A.M. But the studies also show that some cycles and performance efficiency are related inversely. For instance, a pilot can make altitude adjustment more easily at 3:00 A.M. than at 3:00 P.M., even if his efficiency in other tasks is at a low point at 3:00 A.M.

Is there a relationship between body rhythms and health?

It's long been known that among sick people physical distress seems to increase at night; the sick adult wants more pain-killers and the sick child becomes more restive. Fear and loneliness during the night have been blamed. But work with monkeys has shown definite daily rhythmic fluctuations in pain tolerance, which suggest that in humans, too, increased pain at night may be related to body rhythms.

According to experiments in animals, susceptibility to infection is also definitely increased by biologic rhythms. For example, more mice survive injections of the bacteria that cause pneumonia when the injections are given at 4:00 A.M. than when they're given at any other time of day. It appears that rhythmic changes in hormone function or some other aspect of body chemistry influence the infection.

Body rhythms can be upset by sickness. In many cancer patients, body-temperature rhythm is altered. In the emotionally disturbed, there may be changes in sleep rhythm and in secretion of certain chemicals in blood and urine. It may be that specific upsets in rhythms will be found in most, if not all, diseases.

And it now appears that one of the most rewarding aspects of the increasing knowledge of body rhythms will be in the treatment of many diseases.

How are body rhythms useful in treating various illnesses?

There are many examples of how the effectiveness and safety of drugs may be increased by their use in conjunction with body rhythms. Asthmatic children may respond to cortisonelike drugs, but they respond far better when the drugs are given at certain times related to body rhythms. Therefore a little of the drugs at the right time go much further—dosages may be cut and undesirable side effects minimized.

Addison's disease results when the adrenal gland fails to secrete enough hormones. Hormone injections help, but patients seldom feel completely well. Recently, however, doctors have found that if the hormones are taken at strategic times, patients feel better; their extreme fatigue is eliminated.

Researchers have found that if you take aspirin at 7:00 A.M. its effects lasts longer and it can still be detected in the urine twenty-two hours later; taken at 7:00 P.M. it can't be detected beyond seventeen hours.

The duration of effect of a specific dose of a barbiturate may range from fifty to ninety minutes, depending upon the time it is taken. This is also true for stimulants. Some work even suggests that the time of the day when a vaccination is given may determine how effective it will be in providing protection and even possibly in how long the protection will last and whether there will be any undesirable reactions to the shot.

More effective ways to treat emotional problems may be based on timing mechanisms. At the Institute of Living in Hartford, Connecticut, investigators have made laboratory animals anxious by exposing them to fear-inducing situations. And they have found that they have greatest success in extinguishing the anxiety reactions by treating them at the same time of day that the fear was originally induced.

This principle, the investigators believe, may be useful in treating some psychiatric patients. Treatment sessions would not be conducted at random hours but would be scheduled for the same time of day when the patient's original disturbance occurred.

There is some indication now that surgery may be made less dangerous or more effective through consideration of body rhythms. It could be, some investigators believe, that if surgery is scheduled to coincide with the time when a patient's body rhythms are surging upward and are most favorable, the patient might have an easier time during and after the operation.

Recent studies indicate it may be possible to time an X-ray attack on cancer cells during their most vulnerable multiplying phase. Thus the X-rays would be maximally deadly to the cancer cells while doing minimal damage to normal cells, because the rhythms of division differ for cancerous and normal cells.

Can body rhythms be manipulated for good effect?

It's known that some drugs alter rhythms. Some barbiturates, when taken the night before, block the normal morning rise in adrenal hormones. This may explain the hangover effect that sometimes follows use of such drugs.

But it could well be that drugs can be devised to produce desirable changes in body rhythms. And, in fact, body rhythms seem to be related to light and darkness. Therefore, changes in light-dark schedule may be used to produce desirable rhythm changes.

In one experiment with a woman who had a history of menstrual irregularity, a light was left on in her bedroom to simulate moonlight during four nights of her menstrual cycle—the fourteenth, fifteenth, sixteenth, and seventeenth, counting the day of menstruation as the first day. Over a period of several months her previously irregular menstrual cycle became regular, apparently because of the effect of the light. Subsequently, investigators in Boston repeated the procedure with sixteen women and got encouraging results.

There is hope today that light may be used to control ovulation in a way that could make the rhythm method of contraception a practical, reliable technique—a drugless, low-cost, natural method of birth control.

It appears that the study of body rhythms could lead to major breakthroughs in many areas of medicine and psychiatry that would help to overcome and possibly prevent disease and increase longevity. But this is still a very undeveloped area of study.

6

Environment

*Does where one lives have anything to do with
how long one lives?*

Apparently it does. The length of a man's life may depend in
large part on the area of the country in which he lives, according
to a recent study by the National Center for Chronic Disease
Control, a division of the U.S. Public Health Service.

The highest death rate areas lie along the East Coast; areas
west of the Mississippi, particularly in the Great Plains, have the
lowest rates.

In some regions men between forty-five and sixty-four were
found to run a risk of dying twice that of men living in low-rate
areas. For example, the death rate in Scranton and Wilkes-Barre,
Pennsylvania, was about double the rate in south central Nebraska, a region with one of the lowest death rates in the nation.

According to a preliminary study, the pattern of deaths for
women seems to be similarly related to geographical area. And
the areas apparently are much the same for whites and non-
whites.

Is geography related to heart disease?

The death rate patterns for heart disease are generally like
those for all causes. This correlation isn't surprising since more
than half of all deaths occur as a result of heart disease. The

77

Great Plains areas generally have low rates, as do some areas in the Rocky Mountains and also in the mid-South.

In states along the East Coast, the areas of highest death rate for heart disease are nonmetropolitan as well as metropolitan, but elsewhere the peak rate areas tend to be metropolitan. As one extreme example, the heart disease deaths in the state of Nevada occur very largely in the metropolitan area of Reno.

These patterns persist over a period of time; those of recent years are similar to those of twenty and thirty years ago.

While women have heart-disease-connected death rates similar to those of men, they're not identical; the lowest rates more often are in the southern portion of the Great Plains, the highest in the Northeast.

What about cancer?

Some analyses of cancer rates in middle-aged men indicate that the highest death rates are more consistently in metropolitan areas and the lowest more consistently in nonmetropolitan than are the rates for heart disease. There are also substantial similarities, with areas with the highest rates being generally east of the Mississippi River or along the Gulf Coast and the lowest in the Great Plains, Rocky Mountains, and mid-South.

Male death rates for cancer in the United States compare rather favorably with those for other countries. Only one area (Jersey City) has a higher rate than the high Finnish rate, while fifty-four areas in the United States have lower rates than the lowest for any entire country.

Areas with lowest rates of death from lung cancer are generally nonmetropolitan, located in the Rocky Mountains and Great Plains, with some in the mid-South. Areas with the highest rates are nearly all metropolitan and lie in the eastern half of the country. The nonmetropolitan areas with high rates are mostly along or near the Gulf Coast.

What's the geography-disease mystery?

Well, consider cancer. The United States ranks about fourteenth for cancer death rate. But why should it have the third highest leukemia death rate, the lowest for stomach cancer, and a median incidence of breast, uterus, lung, and prostate cancer?

Why should Ireland have a high rate of skin and oral cancers, with ten times the rate of lip cancer of England, only sixty miles away? And why should England have the second highest rate of lung cancer in the world, outdone only by Scotland, very close by, which also has the second highest overall cancer death rate for men? Why should Austria have the highest rate in the world for male cancers, third highest for female? Why should Portugal have the lowest cancer incidence in the world? And why should Israel, next lowest for overall cancer incidence, somehow have the world's highest rate of leukemia for both men and women?

Why chronic disease rates should have geographical patterns not only within a country but throughout the world is a challenging puzzle. The possibility that they may be related, at least in part, to environmental geochemistry—the chemistry of rocks, soils, plants, and water—is being explored.

Are there any striking clues to this mystery?

Water may be a factor in the geographical differences in heart and blood vessel diseases. About a dozen years ago, one investigator turned up inverse correlation between drinking-water hardness and deaths in the United States from hypertensive heart disease: the harder the water, the lower the death rate, and vice versa. After the original U.S. report, some investigators in other countries made similar findings. But others in England and in Sweden found no significant association. Hypertensive heart disease is, of course, caused by severe high blood pressure. Russian investigators said that Moscow (hard water) and Leningrad (soft water) have identical hypertension rates.

Then a distinguished British epidemiologist, Jeremy Morris, presented impressive evidence correlating water hardness and heart disease mortality in regions throughout England and Wales. Confirmatory reports followed from Japan, Canada, the southern United States, and elsewhere.

In British studies covering sixty-one county boroughs with populations of 80,000 or over, the harder the drinking water, the lower the death rate in middle age and early old age. The relationship held true particularly for heart and blood vessel diseases and, to a lesser extent, bronchitis.

Even more recently, British investigators checked on changes in death rates in eleven county boroughs where hardness of the water supply had been substantially changed for a variety of reasons over the past thirty years. They found that the effect on heart-disease-connected death rate was favorable in the towns where water had become harder, unfavorable where it had become softer.

One challenging aspect of heart attacks is the large proportion of sudden deaths from them. In a special study of such sudden deaths, Canadian researchers found they were 20 to 30 percent more frequent in a city that had soft water than in a city that had hard water.

Researchers may have found another clue to the relationship between geography and disease. People living in a rural region on Colorado's eastern plains were found to have a significantly higher risk of developing high blood pressure than people in the rest of Colorado, urban or rural. But this hadn't been true before 1950, and it couldn't be explained by water hardness.

In this case nitrate concentration in the water may be a factor. It is known that explosives workers who handle nitrates have increased risk of hypertension. Investigators think that nitrates in water could increase the risk, too. If this is true, the continuing use of increasingly intensive agricultural methods, particularly the use of nitrogenous fertilizers, could be harmful since they may increase nitrate concentrations in ground water.

What benefits does hard water have?

Water gets its hardness from its content of calcium and magnesium; the more of these two metals, the harder the water is. Studies suggest that these metals may provide some protection against artery disease. The experiments indicate that blood cholesterol levels as well as hardening of the arteries are reduced by calcium and magnesium, possibly because the two metals combine with saturated fats in foods and so reduce the body's assimilation of such fats.

But Dr. Henry Schroeder of Dartmouth Medical School has added a new dimension to the hard-water question. He blames soft water for increased heart disease not because of its lack of calcium and magnesium but because of its high content of cadmium. Schroeder, for one, believes that while hard water lays down a protective lime coating in the water pipes, soft water doesn't; instead, it picks up some carbon dioxide, becomes slightly acid, and, thanks to the slight acidity, it dissolves out and picks up cadium, copper, lead, and other metals from pipes. Cadmium apparently competes with zinc in the body, replacing zinc in activities related to fat utilization. Schroeder feels that cadmium is a key factor in allowing both hardening of the arteries and high blood pressure to develop.

Could it be that traces of metals decide our fate?

This is one of the most provocative areas of medical research today in terms of heart disease and also of other important diseases. The idea is that the body knows how to handle certain metals essential to life. It conserves them when necessary; it gets rid of them when in excess. For example, copper is required for blood formation, and a tiny amount—one-tenth of a gram—stands between human life and death. Man can tolerate an excess of copper up to a point, for a limited amount can be excreted. Beyond this, the excess copper can be poisonous. The same holds for metals the body does not need, such as tin, cadmium, or lead. If these metals enter the body in small amounts, the body can excrete them up to a certain limit. Beyond that limit, symptoms of poisoning appear, as when a painter using white lead paint is affected with painter's colic. Some investigators think that trace metals may prove to be more important factors in human nutrition than vitamins. While the body can make many of the needed vitamins and plants can make all of them, neither man nor plants can produce essential trace metals or get rid of many possibly toxic excesses.

Actually, any significant advances in trace metal research had to wait for the development of microchemical analytical techniques delicate enough to allow researchers to measure the minute metal content of tissue and study tissue responses. Such techniques now permit amounts as low as 50 parts of chromium per *billion* parts of mouse liver to be measured.

How much is known about trace elements?

A lot more is known about their role in agriculture and animal husbandry than about their effects in man. For example, there's a disease in apples that makes them dry and spongy inside; with the addition of just a few spoonsful of boron per acre the disease can be eliminated. When Australia had a problem with sheep becoming swaybacked and feeble, it was solved by the addition of minute amounts of cobalt to salt licks. Just an ounce of cobalt a year keeps 100 sheep healthy.

In animal studies Dr. Schroeder has shown that minute amounts of cadmium can shorten life-span by as much as one-third. And in other studies a trace of chromium added to drinking water—just 5 parts of chromium per million parts of water—made some groups of animals live 20 percent longer.

A puzzling but potentially significant finding in human autopsy studies is that the amount of chromium in tissues declines as people grow older. As compared with newborns, for example, adults have only one-third the chromium level. To determine the significance, Dr. Schroeder completely eliminated chromium from the diet of rats. Within a few months 80 percent had sugary urine, indicative of a diabetic state.

This result ties in with other findings that where chromium levels in tissues are high, diabetes is relatively uncommon; where levels are low, the disease is rampant. Diabetes is a disease caused by insufficient or ineffective insulin; conceivably, insulin is ineffective unless enough chromium is present.

Trace element deficiencies are known to occur in foods. For example, while raw sugar has sizable amounts of chromium, refined sugar contains little or none. Says Schroeder: "Chromium is necessary for the metabolism of glucose. A major source of calories is supplied to us almost free of an element necessary for its metabolism."

Are any other trace metals critical for humans?

Probably many; not necessarily all of them have been determined. Recently investigators have found that zinc promotes healing. When patients with wounds were given oral doses of zinc sulfate, their tissues healed an average of thirty-four days earlier than those of patients who did not receive the zinc compound.

Zinc therapy, some researchers believe, may have some value against atherosclerosis. When oral supplements of zinc sulfate were given to a small group of patients with advanced atherosclerosis, all the patients but one increased their exercise tolerance.

Should trace elements be added to water and food?

Adding trace amounts of certain beneficial metals to our drinking water—just as we now add trace amounts of fluoride to help protect against dental decay—may someday be common practice. One of the most important health research objectives is to determine the healthiest levels for trace metals in water and make certain that these metals are there, adding them if necessary. Tolerance limits for undesirable metals must also be established, and water should be treated to get rid of any excess.

In addition foods could be treated, or the soil in which they're grown. Meantime, because trace elements are present to a greater or lesser degree in various foods, there's a strong argument, as we'll see in chapter 12, for eating not just a balanced diet— balanced for proteins, fats, carbohydrates, vitamins, and the rest —but also a varied diet that includes many different kinds of foods instead of a few. Such variety is most likely to provide suitable quantities of essential trace elements.

Is one area of the country especially healthful?

A stretch of prairie south of the Platte River in Nebraska probably is the most healthful spot in America, particularly for middle-aged men, who have almost one-third less chance of dying of heart disease, stroke, lung cancer, or even of injuries resulting from an automobile accident.

In this area of Nebraska, the weather is extreme. Temperatures fall as low as 29° below zero in winter and shoot up as high as 117° in summer. There are tornadoes, droughts, and hailstorms. Food intake is usually hearty. The men are not toothpicks, but they're rarely obese; the women at most might be considered plump. Smoking is as common as it is elsewhere in the country, and the same holds for drinking. The men look fit, and they do a lot of strenuous hunting.

Some of the residents say it's simply a matter of coming from pioneer stock. But other areas in the country were settled by the same ethnic group and don't have the same health record.

Public health service people who've been observing the area for years still don't have any clear-cut explanation. There might, they think, be something special in the soil, air, or water. Or it could be a geocultural matter—diet, exercise pattern, or just the attitude of life somehow encouraged by this particular stretch of the Great Plains. But they also think it could be a combination of factors, known and unknown, that are peculiar to this area.

Special areas aside, what effects does the stress of urban living have?

Surprisingly, despite what many people assume, the answer is not simple. Our cities have become larger. The 1970 census figures confirm that nearly three-fourths of all Americans now live in and around the sprawling cities. The small town is almost gone. Only 3.3 percent of people live in places with populations of 1,000 to 2,500. The South, traditionally rural, is becoming urbanized at even a faster rate than the rest of the country.

But are Americans suffering increasing stress from overcrowding? Are we, in fact, being increasingly crowded? Not according to the 1970 census; it indicates slightly less crowding. The number of housing units grew a little faster than the population during the 1960–1970 decade. Not so many of us live together as ten years ago. Housing got a bit roomier, too. Most people live in four, five, or six rooms; nearly 5.5 million homes have eight rooms or more, an increase of more than a million in this category in ten years. If a real test of crowding lies in how many people there are per room within a home, that figure has declined. In the great majority of homes there are at least as many rooms as people.

What do studies of crowding effects indicate?

The evidence from animal studies is this: If you crowd animals too much, they suffer in many ways and become vicious, aggressive, and antisocial. This often has been cited as evidence that, for example, high crime rates stem from overcrowding. But, strangely enough, where there's an effort to obtain statistics that really allow valid comparisons—such as studying equal-income groups in both city and country—it becomes apparent that overcrowding in itself does not necessarily make villains of people.

The human race seems to be fantastically adaptable in comparison with other species; hence its success in survival. Humans seem able to adapt to situations, including those of sheer frustration, that would cause breakdowns in animals.

Some recent experiments by investigators from Columbia University and Stanford University show that in short-term conditions of overcrowding, men become more competitive, less lenient, and less disposed to like each other. Under the same conditions, women become more cooperative, more lenient, and more sociable toward one another. Interestingly, the difference existed only when the sexes were kept separate. As soon as men and women were put together in crowded conditions, they behaved just as they would if there were no overcrowding.

Isn't urban life more stressful than rural life?

Actually, in terms of stress, one recent study suggests that urban life may be no worse than rural life.

The seven-year survey of the modernizing experience in Argentina, Chile, East Pakistan, India, Nigeria, and Israel was made by a team of sociologists headed by Dr. Alex Inkeles of Harvard and concluded "Our data . . . decidedly challenge the idea that individuals, merely because they live in cities and work in industry, are less well-adjusted than those living in the countryside and working on farms."

The survey involved comprehensive interviews (lasting up to four hours per person) with 6,000 farmers, industrial workers and other city workers, and migrants newly arrived in cities. All were men between the ages of eighteen and thirty-two. They were questioned about headaches and other health problems, especially those that might be produced by stress. They also had to answer more than fifty questions concerned with "daily life satisfaction."

The results indicated very little relationship between how big and bustling a city was and the psychic adjustments of its workers. In India, boomtown conditions actually produced less stress than conditions in a quiet town.

There was no evidence that factory employment led to increased stress. And the larger and more modern the factory, the less the likelihood of stress symptoms. In addition, the presence or absence of headaches and other psychosomatic symptoms in migrants newly arrived in cities was found to be more closely related to the reward level of the new job than to the mere fact of moving from country to city.

The investigators concluded that the trouble with the common theory that moving to a city causes stress may lie not so much in any wrong view of city life as in a mistaken image of what village life is really like—a kind of idyll that doesn't describe things as they really are.

"The average peasant," says Dr. Inkeles, "suffers deep insecurity both in his relation to nature, whence he looks for his sustenance, and in relation to the powerful figures in his village, be they more powerful peasants, rich landowners, or government officials." In this sense, adds Inkeles, "Traditional village life is not necessarily so different from the life of the simple and poor anywhere else and however dismal urban life and industrial employment may be, moving to them will not necessarily lead to greater psychic distress if the village left behind is not as imagined by the theorists."

Do big cities change people's behavior?

Many studies bear out the stereotype of the mistrustful, unfriendly city resident. In one study, when an experimenter posed as a stranger wishing to use someone's phone, he was admitted three times as often into small-town homes as into city residences.

City people are reputed to be deficient in everyday civilities. People bump into each other and often don't bother to apologize.

They knock over someone's packages and may just mutter something rather than offer to help. Such behavior may be relatively rare in small communities.

But it may not be simply that in cities traditional courtesies are violated. "Rather," believes Dr. Stanley Milgram, a social psychologist, "the cities develop new norms of noninvolvement. These are so well defined and so deeply a part of city life that *they* constitute the norms people are reluctant to violate. Men are actually embarrassed to give up a seat on the subway to an old woman; they mumble 'I was getting off anyway,' instead of making the gesture in a straightforward and gracious way. These norms develop because everyone realizes that, in situations of high population density, people cannot implicate themselves in each others' affairs for to do so would create conditions of continual distraction which would frustrate purposeful action."

Medical World News, a magazine for physicians, not long ago devoted considerable space to the subject. It noted that there have been quite serious suggestions that, as urbanization continues, doctors may find themselves treating more and more psychosomatic and physical effects, ranging from anal itches and rashes that suggest male homosexual activity to the broken arms of children, suggesting child abuse.

It noted, too, that many of the assumptions for this projected unhappy future are based on animal studies. Among other things, researchers have found that when animals are crowded in the laboratory, the sex act, instead of remaining a matter of courtship ritual, becomes just a quick, nervous brutal affair; that homosexuality becomes common even though virtually no mammals in the free state are homosexual; that males brutalize females and females no longer build nests or care for their litters, some of them even killing their young.

It also quoted Desmond Morris, curator of mammals for the Zoological Society of London and author of *The Human Zoo*: "Under normal conditions, in their natural habitats, wild animals do not mutilate themselves, masturbate, attack their offspring, develop stomach ulcers, become fetishists, suffer from obesity, form homosexual pairings, or commit murder." But in zoos, as in urbanized human society, these things occur. "The modern human animal is no longer living under conditions normal for his species. Trapped by his own brainy brilliance, he has set himself up in a huge, restless menagerie where he is in constant danger of cracking."

More recently Dr. Milton Greenblatt, Massachusetts commissioner of mental health, reported to an American Medical Association meeting that overcrowding may play a role in some forms of mental disease. He suggested that man may have specific space needs for his physical and mental well-being and that chronic congestion may produce stresses that make some people unable to cope normally.

But he also noted that to date there have been virtually no investigations to relate crowding in and of itself directly to human disease. While there have been many studies relating population density to mentally induced physical symptoms, neuroses, psychoses, and juvenile delinquency, the studies have not separated crowding from such associated factors as low income, insufficient food, and lack of education.

Does weather influence health?

"A change of weather is sufficient to re-create the world and ourselves," Marcel Proust once remarked. Human reactions to weather are so universally recognized that they even color the language. Such expressions as stormy emotions, tempestuous feelings, cloudy thinking, heated temper, all reflect the belief that weather is a force in life.

The fact is that every time weather elements change the body has to make an adjustment. Most of the time it adjusts easily, almost automatically. At other times weather may make drastic demands, mentally and physically.

Right now, in France, there are efforts to make an exact science, called meteorolopathologie, out of studies of adverse human reactions to weather. And every day now about 1,000 West German physicians phone a private number that gives them a special weather forecast intended to help them care for their patients. A typical forecast, given by the climatology department of the German Meteorological Service, may tell the doctor: "Tomorrow, we expect penetration of humid warm air masses coming from the Mediterranean. It is advisable to pay particular attention to patients with circulatory ailments." German surgeons are among the most frequent users of "medical meteorology." They're concerned about weather conditions on days when they operate, especially when the operations are delicate and can be postponed if conditions are unfavorable. It's known, for example, that hot, humid weather is conducive to hemorrhage.

What kinds of body change does weather produce?

One of the most dramatic changes is the swelling and unswelling of tissues with barometric pressure shifts. If you hold a sponge tightly squeezed in your hand in a pan of water, the sponge will absorb water when you relax pressure, then release the water when you increase pressure. In the same way, studies suggest, body tissues take up more water from the intestinal tract when atmospheric pressure falls—enough to increase leg girth, for example, by an inch within a twenty-four-hour period. Some people may also gain as much as five pounds at such times, as they drink extra fluids to refill the intestinal tract.

Tissue swelling increases pressure within the brain, according to Dr. Clarence A. Mills, a leading medical climatologist who was director of the University of Cincinnati's Laboratory of Experimental Medicine. And since the brain is tightly encased in the bony skull, blood vessels may be squeezed and blood flow diminished, leading to despondency, irritability, and loss of mental acuity. Life becomes rosier and mental acuity rises again when atmospheric pressure rises and extra water is squeezed out of the tissues.

Temperature, too, can have marked effects. The body adjusts to heat and cold by increasing or decreasing sweat gland activity and by moving more blood into or away from the skin. But when heat is prolonged, perhaps for several weeks, further adjustments are needed; the thyroid, adrenals, and other glands become less active so the internal-combustion rate can be reduced and less body heat produced. This means less energy for thinking and acting.

Is it true that some diseases act as weather vanes?

Studies indicate that both gout and sciatica are more painful before a storm. But the classic weather vane disease is arthritis. Although long considered to be an old wives' tale, the weather sensitivity of arthritics—their ability to predict changes because of increased pain at such times—has received some scientific support.

At the University of Pennsylvania Hospital, arthritic patients volunteered to live for periods of two to four weeks in a climate chamber where, without their knowledge, changes could be made in temperature, pressure, humidity, and air movement. When only a single factor was changed, no patient experienced any change in symptoms. But when investigators tried duplicating conditions that precede rainstorms—a drop in barometric pressure along with a rise in humidity—patients complained within a few minutes of increased pain, and their joints became stiff and swollen.

Can weather actually cause disease?

Not directly. But it's believed that weather can so modify body functioning and mental outlook as to weaken resistance to disease. Chilling, for example, lowers body resistance to many diseases. Even in the tropics a sudden decrease in air temperature may be followed by outbreaks of sickness. People who don't adjust their rate of physical activity in high or low temperatures may experience some degree of exhaustion, which may predispose them to disease. Extremely low relative humidity and high winds can fill the air with dust, which irritates breathing passages, increasing susceptibility to infection.

Lung embolism (a lung clot), thrombophlebitis (vein clot and inflammation), and hemorrhage, according to some studies, occur predominantly in warm, damp weather. Migraine, colic, stroke, and epileptic seizures seem to occur more often in cool, damp weather.

Colds and other upper respiratory infections, of course, are more common in winter than in summer—four and a half times more frequent in January, a peak month, than in July. Actually, the bugs that produce the infections are prevalent year-round. But recent studies at the University of Wisconsin by Dr. D. L. Walker show that viruses grow and multiply only over a restricted temperature range. For many viruses that infect man, optimum growing temperature appears to fall about a degree or two below normal human body temperature. Environmental cold might lower body temperature just enough to permit growth of some previously inactive viruses. On the other hand, a rise in body temperature may help to check virus growth, which is possibly the reason why a fever may play some part in choking off infection.

Asthma patients experience an increase in symptoms during sudden drops in temperature. A combination of suddenly rising temperature and falling barometric pressure appears to coincide with an increase in the rate and severity of appendicitis attacks.

One study found an increase in mental hospital admissions coinciding with excessive electrical activity in the atmosphere produced by lightning and sunspots. Theoretically, electric energy in the environment may interact with electrical discharges in the nervous system.

Does weather affect the heart?

Weather can affect the heart, and both the blood and blood pressure as well.

In Holland, while making routine blood pressure checks of normal, healthy Red Cross blood donors, physicians were puzzled to find that the same donors sometimes had pressures 20 percent higher than their usual pressures. They soon established a pattern: during January and February 77 percent of these donors showed elevated pressures. And further studies of a healthy population group found that pressure almost invariably tends to be higher in cold weather, lower in warm.

Weather changes induce blood changes, too. In winter, we have more hemoglobin, the element in red blood cells that transports oxygen. But we also have less gamma globulin, the blood fraction that contains the infection-fighting antibodies. German and Japanese investigators have reported lower blood values for calcium, magnesium, and phosphates in winter; and Swiss workers have found increased resistance in the capillaries, the very tiny blood vessels, in cold weather. Such findings may well be related to health problems.

In very cold weather the heart has to work harder to help maintain normal body temperature. Even people with healthy hearts may feel the strain; there is a tendency to tire more easily. Extremely hot weather increases the flow of blood in the body and places a greater strain on the heart muscle.

Dr. George E. Burch of Tulane University, who has studied climate effects on the heart for twenty years, has found that extreme heat or cold can be especially critical for heart patients. There is pronounced strain during the first days as the body adjusts to new temperature conditions.

While deaths from heart attacks increase in the summer months in subtropical U.S. cities, studies by Burch and Giles show that in northern cities, where summers are relatively mild but the cold weather is severe, the death rate is highest in winter. Burch and Giles point out, however, that 75 percent of the United States has hot and humid weather in summer. Deaths from heart conditions increase greatly in these regions, especially during heat waves. A sudden onset of excessive heat and humidity is particularly threatening to the elderly. But while many die from heat exhaustion and heatstroke, the greatest mortality stems from the effect of heat on heart conditions. When temperature shoots up, the body's effort to maintain its heat-regulation system throws excessive work on the heart, which may be evidenced by an increase in heartbeat rate and intensification of heart murmurs and abnormal heart rhythm.

Burch and Giles found that 65 percent of patients who were being treated successfully for congestive heart failure promptly developed failure again when in hot, humid surroundings. In every case control was reestablished when the patients were placed in a comfortable environment.

Such studies suggest important measures for people with heart problems. They should realize the dangers of heat and humidity. Their outdoor activity should be regulated to avoid particularly hot times of day. The severely disabled should remain especially quiet when heat and humidity are high. Air conditioning may be as essential as proper diet and good nursing care, and they should be wary of moving suddenly from air-conditioned rooms to outside heat.

When air conditioning is not available, large fans should be used. Patients should wear loose, light clothing, and should sponge themselves to facilitate loss of body heat. People with heart conditions should not indulge in hot baths or sunbathing that might be permissible for those with strong hearts.

Is there any merit in the old belief that "a warm winter begets a full cemetery?"

This old adage was popular among early settlers in the United States, but if it once may have been true, it isn't now.

Today, overall mortality is higher in cold winters and hot summers, lower in warm winters and cold summers. But the figures also show marked differences according to age: no seasonal variation at all in mortality in younger people between one and twenty-four years of age, and increased mortality in older people during very cold winters. There is also a tendency for people between ages twenty-five and forty-four to actually thrive under the influence of colder winter temperatures.

That last fact, some researchers believe, may account for the old belief of "warm winter, full cemetery." In the past, when life expectancy was shorter, the twenty-five-to-forty-four age group bulked large in the population. Then, as now, they may have done less well during warm than cold winters. But now, older people are increasingly prevalent in the population as the result of medical triumphs over many severe infectious diseases that once caused early death; thus cold winters produce higher mortality because of their detrimental effects on heart and blood vessel diseases common with age.

What are the most and the least healthful months?

Measured in terms of absence from work because of illness, June is the most healthful month of the year, February the least healthful. On an average day in February, according to one study, 2.65 percent of all workers are home sick.

Studies have indicated that eye and eyelid inflammations are highest in April, lowest in October; middle ear infection is highest in February, lowest in August; earache, highest in February, lowest in June; flu, highest in February, lowest in July; pneumonia, highest in February, lowest in July; sore throat and tonsillitis, highest in January, lowest in July; sinusitis and the common cold, highest in February, lowest in July.

Are there any other physical effects of weather?

Weather apparently influences fertility. Farm animals moved from a temperate climate to the hot tropics become notably slow in reproducing. The same holds true for the human male, according to Dr. E. W. Hartman of the Margaret Sanger Research Bureau. Heat is an effective inhibitor of sperm production. There is evidence, Hartman notes, of a seasonal rhythm of male fertility in this country, with a significant conception drop in the south during summer—by as much as 30 percent in Florida.

Some studies suggest that hot summer weather may affect the intelligence of children born the following winter. During the third month of pregnancy, important brain areas of the fetus are formed; any damage to the fetus at that time may affect the IQ of the child. Such damage may result if a mother reduces her food intake, especially her intake of protein, which she is more likely to do in hot weather than at other times. A study of mental defectives admitted to an Ohio institution over a period of many years found a high percentage born in the first three months of the year (the third month in utero for them was in summer).

Checking pregnancy complications, which also may be associated with mental impairment in babies, investigators in New York City found a significantly higher complication rate in mothers who delivered in winter months.

One English study even suggests that the seasons somehow may influence whether rheumatoid arthritis develops later in life. Incidence of the disease in later life was found to be higher among people born between September and February than among those born between March and August.

Does weather affect one's moods?

Weather can make people excited, blue, lazy, ambitious, nervous, or calm. It's almost as if man were a kind of barometer. Low barometric pressure may produce restlessness and lack of concentration; it may make adults frustrated and quarrelsome, and children irritable. Police records in large cities indicate that more acts of violence, including suicides, occur when barometric pressure falls below 30.00. A 50-year study in one large industrial plant revealed that 74 percent of all lost-time accidents took place when pressure was under 30.00.

Some years ago, in an American Medical Association publication, Dr. Noah Fabricant remarked that Abraham Lincoln was subject to fits of depression, and the blues evaporated when the barometric pressure became stable. "He and his wife, Mary Todd Lincoln," Fabricant wrote, "might have been spared a number of crises in their personal lives had they fully understood the effect of the weather."

Dr. Clarence A. Mills has suggested: "If yesterday's bright idea seems pretty poor today, check the barometer. Knowledge that weather may be the basis of your blues as well as boosting you to your emotional peak can often be of great help in achieving a more tranquil existence. Blame your own and the other person's bad moods on the weather—and rest assured that a change is just around the corner."

Does weather affect the mind?

According to studies by Dr. Ellsworth Huntington, mental function is best at 38° to 40° F as against 64° for physical performance. On standard intelligence tests college students have done only 60 percent as well in summer heat as in winter cold.

Animal experiments underscore the temperature influence. White rats kept at 55° needed only twelve tries before finding the correct path through a maze to a food dish; others kept at 75° needed twenty-eight tries; still others kept at 90° required fifty. A month later, when returned to the maze for a test of memory, those from the 55° room knew the right path immediately; those from the 75° room had to relearn half the steps; the 90° rats had no memory at all.

People often are less mentally efficient in foggy weather than in fair. It used to be a rule in the Bank of England that all important files be locked up on very foggy days because it had been found that clerks keeping the records made a much higher percentage of errors on foggy days.

Apparently, even how well we hear is affected by temperature. Studies at the University of North Carolina suggest that hearing is most keen at 50°. Acuity falls as temperature goes above or below that point.

Do people differ in their responses to weather?

According to Dr. Huntington's studies, where one lives has a considerable influence on one's reaction to change in weather. A person living most of his life in the stable climate of San Francisco, Huntington observed, reacts seventeen times more strongly to weather change than does a person living in the stormy region around Minneapolis. Apparently people used to abrupt and fierce weather swings are more or less inured to change and take it in stride.

Generally, healthy people are much less affected by weather changes than are persons in poor health. It also seems that women endure weather extremes better than men, and they are particularly superior in adapting to cold. Women on the average are smaller in stature and they have less surface area and more fatty tissue insulation; therefore their bodies may be able to conserve heat more efficiently.

What can one do about the weather's effects?

If you have a specific health problem that may be influenced by weather—and one for which air conditioning or possibly another climate might be helpful—medical advice is in order.

When it comes to moving to a different climate for health reasons, other factors may have to be considered. For example, some rheumatoid arthritis patients find a measure of relief in warm, dry areas. But the weather change may not be the only beneficial effect; the relaxation, both physical and emotional, that accompanies trips to such areas may play some role in the relief. If moving permanently to a warm, dry climate introduces emotional upset and financial worry, the arthritic problem may be magnified.

The best bet is to learn to live with the weather. Find out, by keeping a record for a time, the kind of weather that gets you down. Even if you can't avoid it, you *can* take it into account. If you know you're in for an off day or two—and why—you can plan on doing less important jobs, avoiding major decisions, and not driving yourself to frustration since you'll feel better next day or the day after.

It's not a bad idea to check on the influence of weather on spouse and children. You'll probably be relieved to find that many of their black moods are merely responses to weather changes, nothing more.

And you might want to consider this observation made by Dr.

Huntington in his weather studies: Generally, people are at their best in terms of health and energy in November and at their worst in January, February, and March, when they tend to be more tired and susceptible to disease. It's at this tired period that a vacation makes sense. But instead of taking a breather, it's just at this time that many people make ambitious resolutions to work harder. But, if Huntington is right, they're working against nature. "To speed up at the end of January is like taking a tired horse and expecting him to win a race."

What's the difference between weather and climate?

When you watch a TV broadcast showing yesterday's high and low temperatures and how many hundredths of an inch of rain fell, you're considering weather. When you learn that the normal mean temperature in your area for yesterday's date is, say, 68°, and normal rainfall for the current month is three inches, that's climate. In short, weather is what happens today or happened yesterday or may happen tomorrow. Climate is what happens over a long period, the seasonal pattern characteristic of a particular place.

Does city climate differ from country climate?

City air tends to be warmer. City buildings and pavements can store more heat than can grass, leaves, or soil. A city can absorb more sunlight, too. Where much of the sunlight striking the relatively horizontal countryside surfaces is reflected back to the sky, sunlight shining on the city has a good chance of being reflected from horizontal street to vertical building wall and bouncing back and forth, with more of it being absorbed in the end.

The city itself produces large amounts of warmth, especially in winter in the form of heat lost from buildings and generated by vehicles. In summer, air conditioning dumps a lot of heat outside. Where in the country much of the rainfall goes into the ground and a considerable amount is returned to the air by evaporation and plant respiration (both of which absorb heat), in the city much of the rainfall moves into the sewer system and has little cooling effect.

In the city, because of reduced evaporation and warmer temperatures, relative humidity is lower than it is in rural areas. But city rainfall tends to be about 10 percent greater than rural rainfall, mostly the result of drizzly days in the city.

Because of smoke and dust, which on calm days are not blown

downwind but hang overhead and can form fog when conditions are right, cities tend to have about one-third more fog in summer, and 100 percent more in winter.

Have city climates been changing?

There are enough indications that man and his works may be significantly altering city climate to have prompted the National Weather Service to begin a large-scale study of long-term meteorological trends in New York City. The study is expected to help answer such questions as:

1. Is the warming trend being recorded for city temperatures, which runs counter to a worldwide cooling trend, real or a statistical vagary?
2. Is city-generated heat making rain more likely than snow in winter?
3. How much of a braking action do tall buildings have on winds which are needed to keep the atmosphere clean?

Many people scoff at the idea that man can, in this way, make any change in the huge natural forces that create climate. The atmosphere, they point out, weighs more than 5 million billion tons, hundreds of times the weight of all cargo moved throughout the world in a year; nearly the whole of this vast mass is constantly in motion at paces all the way from those of gentle breezes to those of the 200-knot jet stream; and the atmosphere, in addition, is always picking up trillions of tons of water and dumping it hundreds, even thousands, of miles away.

But many scientists believe that delicate natural balances can be upset by man. Once the spread of agriculture was the principal means of man-made change. Now it appears that the spread of cities is more important. As cities grow in population and area and as suburbs become more urbanized, heat concentration increases. This effect could account for the apparent average temperature rise in New York City in recent years.

New York's average annual temperature over an eighty-eight-year period up to 1958 was 53.1°. Since 1958, annual averages have been higher in every year except 1967, when the average was one-tenth of a degree lower. Although differences between the long-term average and averages for recent years amount to only a few degrees, even such small differences could be significant. They mean that the hottest days of summer are even hotter and more people are more uncomfortable.

How does air pollution affect climate?

There is no definitive answer yet. Research has been turning up some contradictory findings. For example, dust particles can reflect radiation away from the earth, thus lowering temperature; but the particles also can absorb and retain radiation, thus raising temperature. Meteorologists must learn a great deal more before they can answer the puzzling questions about air pollution.

Just how big is the air pollution problem?

In recent years in the United States hazardous material has been released into the air at an estimated rate of more than 200 million tons per year, the equivalent of a ton per person. Sources include factories, power plants, municipal dumps, private incinerators, and some 100 million internal-combustion engines. Five categories of pollutants are considered particularly important: carbon monoxide, with about 100 million tons released annually; sulfur oxides, 33.2 million tons; nitrogen oxides, 20.6 million tons; hydrocarbons, 32 million tons; and particulate matter, 28.3 million tons.

What are the ill effects?

Ill effects can come from either high-level, short-term exposure or low-level, long-term exposure.

Exposure to high levels of pollution for a short time can have dramatic, immediate effects. Such exposure occurs when weather conditions are such that a heavy pall of pollution is held over an area for several days. The first episode of high-level exposure that attracted worldwide attention occurred in 1930 in the Meuse River valley in Belgium. In the United States the tragedy in Donora, Pennsylvania, in 1948 crystallized concern: 6,000 of a population of 14,000 became ill and the death rate for a short time soared to ten times the normal rate. In 1952 a five-day episode in London was held responsible for 4,000 deaths.

But low-level, long-term exposure to polluted air has the greater significance. While there may be no immediate increased death rate, low-level exposure over an extended period can lead to slow development of deleterious conditions, giving rise to chronic diseases of several types and impairment of body defenses.

For example, atmospheric pollutants such as sulfur oxides,

nitrogen oxides, and ozone can inactivate or even destroy cilia, the hairlike structures in the breathing passages that normally help sweep away impurities and debris. Sensitive underlying cells are left unprotected, and they may enlarge or attempt to regenerate excessively, thus narrowing the respiratory passages and making breathing more difficult. Moreover, irritants may stimulate production of increased or thickened mucus which, without cilia to propel it outward, collects foreign matter, including bacteria and other microorganisms. As a result respiratory infections develop more easily and are less readily overcome.

Swelling of cells in the air passages due to pollutants, combined with spasm or involuntary contraction of the muscles surrounding the air passages, may lead to chronic bronchitis, emphysema, and asthma. In recent years in the United States chronic bronchitis and emphysema have become the most rapidly increasing causes of death.

Very recent work by Dr. Arian Zarkower of Pennsylvania State University suggests that sulfur dioxide and other air pollutants can interfere with the body's production of antibodies that combat disease organisms.

For more than ten years, Dr. Warren Winkelstein, Jr., of the University of California School of Public Health has compared the health of people living in poor areas where industrial pollution is dense with the health of people living in wealthier, relatively pollution-free neighborhoods. He found that the overall death rate was twice as high in the polluted areas, and the death rates from tuberculosis and stomach cancer in particular were three times as high.

Relatively low levels of nitrogen oxides have been linked to children's susceptibility to Asian flu. Studying students at Stanford University, Dr. William H. Durham and other investigators recently found that the incidence of colds, sore throat, and gastrointestinal flu increases on warm, sunny days, when air pollution levels tend to be higher than on windy or rainy days.

Increased carbon monoxide levels have been linked with increased likelihood of motor vehicle accidents and with decreased survival of patients experiencing heart attacks and those with cirrhosis of the liver. Exposure to carbon monoxide in amounts no greater than 10 parts per million parts of atmosphere (not uncommon in many cities) for about eight hours has been shown to impair mental performance because of reduced ability of blood to carry enough oxygen to the brain. (Carbon monoxide usurps the place of oxygen in the blood.)

It's commonly said in medical as well as lay circles that the rise in cancer and other chronic diseases may simply be related to the longer life-span today, a result of medical progress. In other words, people live longer and have more opportunity to develop chronic disease. But Dr. John J. Hanlon, assistant surgeon general of the U.S. Public Health Service says "This is a gross oversimplification. Chronic and degenerative physical and mental ailments have increased, probably in large part because of environmental changes which have resulted from extensive and ever-increasing industrialization and urbanization."

According to Dr. Paul Kotin, director of the National Institute of Environmental Health Sciences, man's misuse of the environment is costing Americans $35 billion a year because of ill health and related losses. Of the nation's total health bill of about $70 billion a year, $7 billion goes for treating illnesses resulting from the environment. In addition, he figures, Americans lose $25 billion annually through lost wages and services attributable to environmentally caused illnesses. The rest of the $35 billion consists of costs of compensation and rehabilitation for people whose illnesses are largely attributable to environmental factors.

If one recent medical review is right, at the very least even just a halving of air pollution levels could reduce bronchitis morbidity and mortality by 25 percent and possibly by as much as 50 percent; could save one-fourth of all lives now being lost to lung cancer; could avoid one-fourth of the sickness and deaths due to respiratory diseases; and could reduce heart disease sickness and death rates by 20 percent and the overall incidence of cancer by 15 percent.

Does air pollution affect our emotions?

It seems to. A Connecticut physician, Dr. Marshall Mandell, recently has reported finding what he considers to be direct cause-and-effect relationships between air pollutants and various neurological and psychological disorders usually considered to be emotional in nature. When he placed patients in a controlled environment, then introduced various pollutants, he found that the pollutants promptly precipitated epileptic seizures, depression, anxiety, and stammering—all symptoms of which the patients had complained earlier.

According to Dr. Alfred Strickholm, an Indiana University psychologist, pollution may have subtle effects responsible for some of the uglier character traits of modern man: "Chronic high irritability, possibly affecting our whole society, is an example of what I'm talking about. Society may be suffering from subtle sickness to which pesticides and other pollutants are contributing. People can be sick all the time and not know it. They can feel run-down, chronically bad, and think it's normal."

Is air pollution mostly confined to large metropolitan areas?

No. It's estimated that every community in this country with a population of more than 50,000 has a sufficient concentration of sources of air pollution to produce adverse effects on human health. A recent report to the New York State Medical Society noted: "We know that air quality can be low in many of our smaller and rural communities as well. We know that less than lethal levels of air pollution can foul our skies, irritate our eyes and lungs, and damage our homes and properties. Even though final and definite answers are not available, we are also aware that research has implicated long-term exposure to lower levels of air pollution to a host of debilitating physical ailments."

What about the other hazards that affect us?

Pesticides, which eventually end up in our water sources, are of concern. By now, the body fat of the average American contains 12 or more parts per million of DDT and lesser amounts of several other pesticides. So far, except for some accidental deaths in children and crop dusters exposed to very large amounts, these substances have not been proved harmful to humans in smaller quantities, but there is no guarantee they may not be in the long run. We've been exposed to them only since World War II, which is a relatively short time as such things go.

Another source of concern is the 3.5 billion tons of waste material discarded annually in the United States—165 million tons of household wastes, 200 million tons of municipal and industrial wastes, 2 billion tons of agricultural wastes, and over a billion tons of mining wastes. A significant amount of it contaminates our water supply by runoff or direct discharge.

Is it possible for hazards to interact?

There's increasing evidence of the complex effects of combinations of some hazards. For example, a habitual cigarette smoker has about ten times the risk of dying of lung cancer as a nonsmoker. An asbestos worker has seven to ten times greater risk of dying of lung cancer.

But the combined risk of cigarette smoking and working with asbestos is not just the sum of the two risks, seventeen to twenty times greater risk; rather the risk is eighty to ninety times greater. If substantial and prolonged exposure to automotive air pollution is added, the risk is again multiplied several times.

How serious is the noise pollution problem?

"A stench in the ear," Ambrose Bierce called noise many years ago, talking simply from the standpoint of a sensitive, thinking man. Now noise is considered a medical and health problem of prime importance.

A bizarre medical case was reported recently by Dr. A. J. Philipzoon, chief of the Ear, Nose and Throat Clinic at the University of Amsterdam. "A man 82 years old . . . had the complaint of bad hearing. . . . During the last years he became progressively deaf, and for that reason he consulted our department whether it was possible to get a hearing aid.

"At the examination we found a normal eardrum of the right ear. In the left ear we found much cerumen [wax]. The 'cerumen' proved to be a dirty piece of cotton wool which had obstructed the ear canal completely. When we asked how this plug had come into his ear, the patient became very angry and told us that when he had an otitis [ear infection] thirty-two years ago, the family doctor had left a plug of cotton wool in his ear. Although the patient had told the doctor that in his opinion there was still a plug left in his ear, the latter had told him this was not true. Thus nothing happened for thirty-two years!"

After the cotton plug was removed, Philipzoon tested hearing and was struck by the findings. In the right ear, he found pure deafness; in the left ear hearing was far better. In his opinion, the plug of cotton had functioned as an ear defender for thirty-two years.

We need such defense today. We're being bombarded by noise, and according to recent research, noise pollution may be just as dangerous as other pollution, and not limited just to hearing impairment.

How high do noise levels run in our world today?

One decibel is about the level of the weakest sound that a person with good hearing can pick out in a quiet location. At a distance of five feet, a soft whisper registers about 30 decibels. In normal conversation the human voice is almost 70; a blaring radio, 110; a symphony concert at its loudest, 130; a turbojet can reach 160. Definite ear discomfort occurs at about 120 decibels. At 140 there is outright pain.

According to the U.S. Environmental Protection Agency, the overall loudness of environmental noise has been doubling every ten years. The average noise polluting our environment today, some studies indicate, has come close to reaching 85 decibels, which is the highest level considered safe for the ears. But "average" means that sometimes the level is below and some-times it's above 85 decibels. Many industries now protect em-ployees against chronic noise levels above 85 decibels.

Even in secluded vacation areas, the noise of minibikes and snowmobiles and sounds from transistor radios disturb what was once beautiful silence. The din in the home is considerable, with the kitchen probably ranking as the noisiest room thanks to a variety of sound-producing appliances which emit up to 100 decibels.

Traffic and other city noises approach or even exceed the danger level. In the city one is beleagured by noises from honk-ing cars, wailing police and fire engine sirens, riveting, jack-hammers, air compressors, pile drivers, and garbage trucks.

When is hearing damaged?

"We do not know how much exposure to these intense city noises will cause hearing loss, but the danger is there," says Dr. Samuel Rosen of the Mount Sinai Medical School, in New York City, who ranks as one of the country's most distinguished ear specialists.

Rosen recently studied 1,500 Mabaan tribesmen of East Cen-tral Africa. He was interested in finding out whether the prevail-ing theory that human hearing degenerates naturally with age is valid. He found that the tribesmen had remarkably acute hear-ing even at age 80. The reason, he believes, lies in the tribe's noiseless, pastoral environment.

Examinations of teen-agers who had exposed themselves to loud music in discotheques where the noise levels measured 90 to 100 decibels with frequent peaks of 120 decibels, revealed temporary 40 percent loss of hearing in 10 percent of youngsters and lesser temporary hearing loss in another 80 percent.

At the Central Institute for the Deaf in St. Louis, researchers exposed animals to brief periods of above-normal noise levels and found that they developed swollen membranes within the ears.

What are the other unhealthy effects of noise?

At Stanford Research Institute, brain-wave patterns of sleeping subjects have been found to be radically changed by sound levels that do not awaken them. Loud noises cause blood vessels to constrict, the skin to pale, and the muscles to tense and trigger the release of adrenal hormones into the bloodstream with a consequent increase in nervousness and tension.

Animal studies—at the University of California Medical School, the University of Montreal, the University of Western Australia, and elsewhere—have shown that loud noises make animals susceptible to virus infections, interfere with kidney function, encourage gastric ulcers, and even increase the rate of tooth decay.

And there is also mounting evidence of an unhealthy effect of noise on the heart. In Europe, where investigation of noise has long been under way, many researchers believe that the heart is subjected to abnormal strain from noise above the 90-decibel level. Using special instrumentation, Salvatore Maugeri of Pavia University in Italy finds that such sounds produce a generalized spasm of arteries.

Dr. Meyer Friedman, a leading heart investigator in San Francisco, studied the effect of excessive noise on blood fats of rats and rabbits, and found that it doubled the triglyceride level in rats and increased the cholesterol level in rabbits significantly.

Dr. Rosen, looking for some connection between noise and heart ailments, conducted an experiment in two mental hospitals in Finland. Patients at one hospital were fed a diet rich in saturated fats; patients at the other were fed a diet almost entirely free of fats. Over several years, those at the second hospital developed far less heart disease than those at the first. Surprisingly, their hearing also improved. When the diets were reversed, hearing and heart disease trends reversed, too. Coupling these findings with those of other researchers on noise, Rosen concluded that noise, hearing, and heart disease are interrelated and that noise is a contributor to heart disease as well as hearing loss.

It appears that extreme noise may even produce mental illness. British investigators recently reported a study covering two years of admissions to a psychiatric hospital, showing a significantly higher admission rate from a maximum noise area around London's Heathrow Airport than from outside it.

What can be done about excessive noise?

Plenty. During the reign of Queen Elizabeth I of England, a strict law forbade wife beating during the night. The legislative idea wasn't to emancipate women—wife beating was permitted during daylight hours—but simply exemplified a sixteenth-century effort to deal with noise.

Today, according to the Environmental Protection Agency, noise differs from most other environmental pollutants in one important aspect: the necessary knowledge and technology are available to control almost every indoor or outdoor noise problem. Construction equipment, planes, street traffic, subways, air conditioners, office machines—all these and many more sources of high-level noise can be made quieter through proper engineering techniques.

Says Dr. Rosen: "Acoustical science and technology have provided the army with an inaudible motor for front-line use, the navy with silently operating submarines, and the air force with an almost silent plane. Surely some of the same techniques applied to civilian use would do much to alleviate the health hazards of excessive noise. Public pressure could help bring about legislation and its enforcement."

Would these measures be costly?

Some noise control measures might be expensive, but certainly not all of them. The Environmental Protection Agency reports that one manufacturer, for example, has developed a garbage truck reported to be 60 percent quieter than those in common use, and the additional cost is only $100 per truck.

At some increase in cost, but not necessarily prohibitive increases, power generators can be quieted with baffles and sound-absorbing materials; auto tires can be made with quieter treads; noise control can be built into the design of other equipment and machinery.

New vibratory pile drivers and jackhammers have been developed to operate with relatively little clatter; noise screens can be used for blasting operations; subway and elevated structures can be acoustically treated.

Few cities in this country have as yet included noise control requirements in building codes, though this is common practice in European countries. Plastic plumbing pipes, for example, are quieter and even cheaper than copper or lead pipes but are seldom used because of code restrictions.

Actually, many experts believe that technology can handle most noise problems at relatively moderate cost. But even if only a small increase in the price of an article results from reducing its noise output, a manufacturer may hesitate to make the improvement unless he can be assured that his competition will do the same. Legal controls may be needed to assure this.

7

Work, Income, and Social and Marital Status

Can success kill?

Go ahead and be as successful as you wish. There's a common idea that people who get ahead and achieve distinction must sacrifice their health in the process. That's not necessarily true at all.

Not long ago, prompted by articles in business publications indicating conflicting opinions about the longevity of successful men, life insurance company analysts made a study of 6,329 prominent professional and business men listed in *Who's Who in America*. They found that on the average these men live longer than men in the general population.

From age forty-five on, the distinguished men had a death rate 30 percent below that of white men in the general population. And when compared to men in similar occupations who had not achieved prominence, the successful men had a 40 percent lower death rate.

It is particularly noteworthy that the eminent men enjoyed the greatest (most favorable) disparity in mortality at ages fifty to fifty-nine, contradicting an old belief that the mercilessness with which men drive themselves during their forties to achieve outstanding positions is reflected in broken health when they are in their fifties.

106

Were there any variations by occupation?

Yes. In the *Who's Who* group, those with death rates close to the average for the group as a whole were business executives, judges, lawyers, engineers, artists, illustrators, and sculptors. Doing better than average were clergymen and church officials, educators, military men—and doing best of all were scientists. On the other hand, outstanding physicians and surgeons and government officials had a slightly higher mortality than the average. The highest mortality was for correspondents and journalists and, to a lesser degree, authors, editors, and critics.

The business executives listed in *Who's Who* made a very strong showing when compared with the total U.S. white male population. At ages forty-five and over, they had a mortality only 71 percent of that for other men. In the forty-five-to-sixty-four age range their mortality was only 48 percent of that for all white businessmen at corresponding ages.

The educators—college presidents, deans, administrators, professors—had a mortality rate 38 percent lower than all white males in the general population.

For judges and lawyers listed in *Who's Who*, mortality was one-fourth less than for all white males and 30 percent less than for judges and lawyers at all levels of accomplishment.

While men of letters—authors, writers, critics, historians, editors, correspondents, and journalists—had the highest mortality rate among the eminent men, it was still 10 percent less than for all white men in the general population.

Medical men of prominence didn't do as well as the general average of prominent men—at ages forty-five to sixty-four their death rate was 20 percent higher—but still they had a mortality of 22 percent less than for all white males in the general population.

Churchmen of *Who's Who* distinction had a mortality only 87 percent of that for all the prominent men and only 62 percent of that for all white males. And distinguished scientists had a death rate 79 percent of that for all prominent men and 55 percent of that for all white men.

But doesn't the stress of success imperil the heart?

The "executive heart" myth—the belief that successful men in business die of heart disease more often than others do—is all but abolished by the *Who's Who* study.

In addition, a national study covering 270,000 men in one

huge American industry found that men who rise to the top are no more susceptible to heart disease than are men who fail to work their way into the executive suite. In fact, the executives have fewer heart attacks than others.

This investigation was made by a team headed by Dr. Lawrence E. Hinkle of Cornell University Medical College, who collected data over a five-year period on 270,000 men working for the Bell System, the link of telephone companies stretching coast to coast. The age, educational level, occupational category and level, and the past career and medical conditions of almost all the men employed by the twenty-eight Bell System operating companies were tabulated. Over this period, all illness and deaths due to coronary disease—6,347 cases—were investigated.

The results were surprising. At all ages from thirty-five to sixty-four, heart attack rates for managers and executives were lower than for workmen and foremen. Even the most rapid advancement—to a managerial or executive position before age forty-five—was associated with a rate no higher than that of workmen and foremen of the same age and length of service. Executives of all ages experienced only 60 percent of the expected incidence of heart disease.

Transfer from one Bell System unit to another in a distant location, which might impose stress, also had no effect on heart-disease incidence.

In contrast, though, education background turned out to have a striking effect. Among college men the incidence of disabling coronary disease was 30 percent lower than among noncollege men. Hinkle tried to learn the reason. The findings suggested that the differences in education apparently reflect differences in social and economic background. College men proved to be consistently taller and slimmer than noncollege men of the same age and job level. Presumably, family background and early health and nutritional experience play a role.

College men also begin to smoke later in life and are less likely to smoke at all. By age fifty-five, there were nearly twice as many cigarette smokers among the noncollege men. Also, college men in general tend to take better care of themselves physically.

But some critics of the Bell study point out that the subjects were all company men in a closed shop, and these men were almost assured of salary increases. The critics point to a study on the West Coast contrasting 800 oil, bank, and insurance executives employed by large companies with 800 physicians, most of whom were self-employed. Over a twenty-year period, twice as many of the doctors had heart attacks.

Do any studies relate job stress and heart disease?

Some years ago, Dr. Henry I. Russek, a New York cardiologist, observed that among 100 young coronary patients, emotional stress related to their jobs seemed significant. At the time of their attacks, 91 percent were holding down two jobs, working more than sixty hours per week, or experiencing unusual fear, insecurity, discontent, frustration, restlessness, or feelings of inadequacy in relation to their work.

Russek went on to study 14,000 people in fourteen categories of jobs, with the jobs rated according to their possible stressfulness. When, for example, security traders and security analysts in the forty-to-sixty-nine age group were compared, coronary attacks were found to be more than twice as prevalent among the traders as among the analysts. The traders are believed to work under more stressful conditions. Similarly, when general practitioners who may be under more stress were compared with dermatologists and pathologists, who may be under less stress, the general practitioners were found to have three to four times the number of heart attacks experienced by the specialists.

It also turned out that trial lawyers had three times as many attacks as patent attorneys and real estate lawyers, again presumably because of the stressful nature of the work of trial lawyers.

But stress is probably a part of almost every job. A nationwide study by the University of Michigan's Institute for Social Research found indications of widespread job stress. One-third of all employees interviewed in this study complained that they had no clear idea of their responsibilities; 48 percent said they often felt caught in the middle between people demanding different things of them; and 45 percent complained of being overloaded with work.

So, is stress a killer or not?

Many researchers are convinced that the response to stress, not the stress itself, can be harmful—that it is a matter of personality. An imperturbable tycoon may take in stride the most severe kind of stress, while a nervous person could suffer a coronary episode even in a placid job such as assistant librarian.

Dr. Herman K. Hellerstein of Western Reserve University in Cleveland has spent many years studying the actual heart stresses encountered in industry and in the more stressful occupations. He has monitored TV broadcasters and entertainers, advertising men, trial lawyers, sky divers, and surgeons for long periods, using sophisticated instruments, including portable electrocardiograph equipment. He sought answers to such questions as: Is a TV newscaster's heart affected by the pressure of deadlines? What are the heart stresses on a lawyer in the heat of a courtroom argument? What are the strains on the surgeon confronted by an emergency in the operating room and required to make crucial split-second decisions?

The results were surprising. Hellerstein found that few test subjects showed any really great heart response to job stress situations. The widely held idea that deadlines and decision making put a burden on the heart was not upheld. The average heart rate during the working period in TV studios was no greater than that in a mill or a factory. Despite the drama of the operating room, the average rise in blood pressure for thirty-nine surgeons was only fifteen points. The working pulse for surgeons averaged 104 beats a minute. Some surgeons even had a drop in pulse rate when they entered the operating room, suggesting that they had done their worrying prior to entering and once inside concentrated on their work.

Occasionally, critical moments in the operating room did produce a rise in pulse rate. One surgeon with a steady reading of 90 had a fleeting reading of 130 when a tube from a heart-lung machine slipped out of a patient's vein.

The study provided some fascinating insights. For example, Hellerstein monitored a surgeon through two operations, one a simple hernia repair, the other an exploratory operation on a young girl. The peak heart rate for the surgeon came during the hernia repair. The reason was that the young girl was found to be suffering from inoperable cancer when opened up and the surgeon, unable to proceed, felt compassion but no challenge, anger, or guilt. The hernia repair, however, required alertness and skill.

Throughout one operation, an anesthesiologist had a pulse rate in the 90s, but an hour later his reading jumped to 125 while he was discussing a malpractice suit with his lawyer.

A very busy internist was monitored by Hellerstein to learn the effect on the heart of a heavily overloaded daily work schedule. The internist had several examination rooms going at the same time, his phone rang constantly, he was often confronted with difficult decisions. During the monitoring, for example, he found a case of lung cancer. But his heart rate and blood pressure remained normal. Once, however, during the forty-eight-hour study period, the doctor's heart rate did shoot up: when he had to talk by phone with a hospital official. Between physician and official there existed overt hostility.

The pressures of deadlines and heavy responsibilities do not necessarily put stress on the heart, Hellerstein concludes. The personality of the individual and his specific response to job and stress are more significant than the job and stress themselves. As we'll see in chapter 8, extensive studies indicate that there is a definite personality type for heart attacks.

Is there any danger in "moving up in the world?"

There could be. Dr. S. Leonard Syme, professor of epidemiology at the University of California at Berkeley has made some interesting observations. One is that men have increased risk of developing coronary heart disease when, as adults, they live in situations different from those in which they were reared. In one study, men who grew up on farms and moved to the city as adults to take white-collar jobs had a coronary heart disease rate three times higher than a comparable group of men who remained on the farm. On the other hand, men from farm backgrounds who moved to the city but took blue-collar jobs showed no significant increase in risk.

"There is a suggestion," Syme believes, "that risk increases when men 'move up in the world'—when they grow up learning one set of rules to live by, only to end up in another world where other rules are necessary."

A second observation is that men run increased risk of coronary disease when, during their adult lives, they undergo frequent changes in life situation. In two studies, men with frequent changes of job or residence had coronary rates two to three times higher than those of men who had fewer changes.

A third observation is that men have increased risk when they live in urban, industrialized areas. In a North Carolina study, changes in coronary heart disease mortality were analyzed in a large number of rural communities that slowly became urbanized. A much higher death rate was noted among the original residents of those towns that had grown in size; the original residents were stable but the world about them changed.

In such examples, Syme suggests, the risk of developing coronary heart disease seems to increase when men "are faced with challenges for which they have no ready-made, tried and tested, group-sanctioned solutions. A person plunged into a world for which he is not prepared wonders what the proper 'rules of the game' are, wonders who he is, and where he is going, and why."

Is work satisfaction a favorable influence on health and longevity?

Yes, according to data compiled during a recent thirteen-year study at Duke University Medical Center. Dr. Erdman B. Palmore studied 270 volunteers between sixty and ninety-four years of age, examining the relative importance of physical, mental, and social factors in predicting longevity. He found that men and women who were happy with their work (whether paid employment or household activities) lived longer than those who were unhappy with their jobs.

Palmore devised a concept called the "longevity quotient" (LQ). The LQ is the number of years an individual survives from a given point in time (in this case his examination date when he entered the study) divided by the expected number of remaining years of life at that time as predicted by the usual actuarial tables based on age and sex alone. An LQ of 1.0 means a person lived exactly as long as expected; an LQ greater than 1.0 means he lived longer than expected; and an LQ less than 1.0 means he died before expected. For example, if a man lived fifteen years after the examination and had an actuarial expectancy of only ten years, his LQ would be 1.5, meaning that he lived half again as long as was expected.

Palmore found that such factors as smoking and physical functioning, which would logically play an important role in determining longevity, were less important than the work satisfaction rating. If an individual's work satisfaction was low, his life-span was predicted to be shorter—and the prediction usually proved true.

As an example, an eighty-one-year-old man in the study had average health and, according to actuarial tables, a remaining life expectancy of 5.6 years. But his work satisfaction rating, even at that advanced age, was the highest possible. Using Palmore's guide, he was expected to survive 9.5 years. He lived another 11.6 years, more than double the actuarial prediction but reasonably close to that of the LQ.

"We know that the mind affects the body in various ways," says Palmore. "We don't completely understand why, but we can see further evidence from this study that a relationship exists between the mental state of the person and his physical condition."

Can ways be found to make work more satisfying?

Some efforts are being made in this direction. For example, in Cologne, West Germany, men and women at the Lufthansa head-quarters and at many other offices and factories go to work when they want to and stay as long as they want to, within reason. As reported by *The New York Times,* "This fast-spreading arrangement is being hailed by those who have tried it as a blessing to employers and employees alike."

The workers still have to account for their total work hours. But the fact that each can work according to his peak produc-tivity patterns (the "morning" people who are at their best early in the day coming in early, the "afternoon" people coming in later) means their output in fewer hours is greater than it would be during longer hours that include their hours of lowest effi-ciency.

Reportedly at Lufthansa 95 percent of employees find the system helpful. And because they are "very happy with the in-dividual freedom they have," says a Lufthansa executive, "we find it much easier to recruit now."

Unfortunately, such a flexible system isn't geared, at least not yet, to assembly lines or some service industries. But at least two Swedish automobile manufacturers, Volvo and Saab, have begun to eliminate the assembly line in favor of team production methods. The idea is to take a step toward reducing the "de-humanizing" effects of factory life by having parts brought to cars to be installed by semiautonomous groups of workers rather than transporting cars through long lines of men, each per-forming a single monotonous job. Whether or not this effort works out, it illustrates a growing concern over low worker morale, which may be reflected in absenteeism, poor work, and hostility.

Also indicative of that concern was the holding of a special symposium, "Technology and the Humanization of Work," at a recent annual meeting of the American Association for the Advancement of Science. A major theme was that modes of work that may have been acceptable in the past are increasingly oppressive to young workers in factories and offices. There must be efforts to find ways of overcoming monotony and improving human relations to make work more satisfying.

Some American companies have begun to experiment with what is called "job enrichment." Basically, as reported by the *Wall Street Journal,* "job enrichment" means letting workers plan and control more of their work as a way to challenge them, make their jobs more interesting, and increase their productivity.

For example, American Telephone & Telegraph encourages subsidiaries to give repairmen greater autonomy and make each responsible for maintaining all phones in entire neighborhoods. Chrysler has begun to involve workers in departmental decisions. At one of its plants, General Electric gives machine operators a greater role in scheduling work and devising work rules.

The job enrichment concept is young and controversial. There is some question about how well it will work out on a broad scale, but at least it's getting a trial.

What about job safety? Aren't a lot of people killed while doing hazardous work?

Of course some work carries an extra risk of death. But generally there has been a considerable reduction in the extra mortality as industry has adopted more effective safety precautions and preventive measures.

For example, over the past forty years death rates for laborers in general construction have come down from 229 percent above that for standard insurance risks to 119 percent above. Similarly, above-average mortality rates for freight handlers, section and track workers, yard workers, and other railroad industry unskilled workers has dropped from 177 to 137 percent. For unskilled workers in metals smelting, refining, and founding plants the rates have fallen from 235 percent above average to 153 percent.

Men in the metal manufacturing industries—electroplaters, grinders, buffers, polishers, metal chippers—also now have reduced mortality rates. Much of the improvement stems from new operating procedures and better equipment that offers increased protection against harmful dusts, fumes, and other hazards.

Mortality rates for anthracite miners have declined sharply, but those for bituminous coal miners have changed very little. Accidents have been responsible for more than a third of the deaths among all underground coal miners. Death rates from respiratory diseases among miners have also been high.

In occupations that have shown a relative increase in mortality, accidental deaths are a major cause of this increase. For example, among truck drivers whose mortality has gone up from 112 to 151 percent over that for standard risks, accidents account for three out of ten deaths, and the accidental death rate for truck drivers is running 10 percent higher than a generation ago.

There is plenty of room for job safety improvement. Official figures of the Bureau of Labor Statistics show that 14,500 people are killed on the job each year. (That figure can be compared with 14,950 murders in the nation each year.) Furthermore, about 2.2 million people in the work force of 75 million suffer disabling injuries that cause them to lose time from work. Some recent estimates put the disabling injuries higher by about 8 percent. And there is some belief that serious injuries not causing a significant loss of time from the job might be as high as 25 million a year, or about ten times the presently reported figure.

An occupational health survey by the Institute of Medicine of Chicago covering 803 plants in the Chicago area found that 28 percent had serious health hazards. A projection of the figures to the estimated 14,453 plants in the area would indicate that more than 4,000 plants, employing 484,827 workers, require "further industrial hygiene evaluation."

Under the Occupational Safety and Health Act of 1970, nearly all industries, including those with only one employee, are required to provide safe places of employment free of health hazards. And new standards for industrial health are to be established from the research and recommendations by the National Institute of Occupational Safety and Health. These standards will cover exposure to such things as lead, asbestos, silica, cotton dust, carbon monoxide, mercury, heat stress, noise, ultraviolet radiation, and other potentially harmful factors. Employers are expected to comply with standards and will be subject to unannounced inspections.

Is retirement a ticket to the mortuary?

Retirement seems to sound the death knell for some people, but certainly not for all. When a man who has few or no interests outside his work retires he can fall apart. It's not simply a matter of his idleness weighing on him; he lacks identity.

There's a lot of talk about preparation for retirement, including financial planning and possibly style-of-living adjustment. But more essential in terms of health is long-term preparation in another sense: the development of interests useful and intriguing enough so that retirement can be a time anticipated as an opportunity to pursue those interests on a larger scale.

Is there such a thing as too much work?

Sure. And although overwork is not healthful, there are "workaholics," people with "the uncontrollable need to work incessantly." That definition is offered by a psychology of religion professor, Wayne E. Oates, in his book *Confessions of a Workaholic*.

Himself an ex-workaholic, Oates says that the workaholic virtually drops out of the human community and eats, drinks, and sleeps his job. Every morning he is up at a set hour; at his office he is "merciless in his demands upon himself for peak performance" and "without qualms about telling off both high and low" when their work is sloppy. Arriving home late, he heads for his study "to make the best of the remaining hours of the day," unable to differentiate between plain loyalty and compulsive overcommitment to his employers.

There are many motivations for becoming a workaholic. Drudges sometimes are those who have guilty feelings over pleasure. The workaholic also may have fantasies of being omnipotent, imagining that only he can do what needs doing. He also may enjoy, consciously or not, making others uncomfortable by accomplishing more than they do. It's hardly a rewarding or healthy life.

What about the saying, "Hard work never killed anyone?"

As medical men point out, nobody can go on working virtually all the time with little or no recreation and not upset the autonomic nervous system. The autonomic is the part of the nervous system that takes care of needs and functions automatically, without any thought on the part of the individual. The autonomic system functions best when there is a pattern of satisfying work *and* restorative leisure. When the work pattern is too long and strenuous (whether it's mental, physical, or both), the autonomic system rebels and the result can be fatigue, irritability, or even real sickness. Any or all of these may upset relations with family, friends, and fellow workers, leading to tensions that make the situation worse.

Says one physician: "Unless the victim of this problem is driven to overwork by harsh economic necessity, the solution is not only plain to see but easy to carry out; work should be moderated and relaxation increased. Relaxation, of course, means different things to different people. Travel may appeal to the office worker and a quiet stay at home to the traveling salesman; the easy chair to the laborer and vigorous sport to the sedentary craftsman. But the common denominator is contrast and the goal is refreshment."

Obviously, there are times when extra work is needed to meet debts incurred by sickness in the family or children's educations, or simply to meet a job deadline. Such temporary extra exertion isn't likely to hurt a healthy, well-adjusted person who intends, once the need is met, to go back to a more balanced routine.

Is there anything one can do about easing job tensions?

Job tensions are experienced at some point by everyone—from the janitor to the chairman of the board. It helps, first of all, to look at tensions in proper perspective.

A certain amount of tension and fretting about job responsibilities, office politics, bosses, subordinates, deadlines, and all the rest isn't going to do any harm. In fact, a certain amount of tension might even be considered normal. Many people work better under tension. Tension can even be pleasurable; witness your feelings when watching a suspenseful movie.

Most people handle tension in everyday life without trouble. The tense feelings, even if unpleasant, usually pass without harm.

It's when tension doesn't pass, when it builds up, that it may become harmful. Do you find yourself getting hopping mad at slight irritations, such as traffic delays, stuck desk drawers, recalcitrant locks? Do you gulp meals, smoke more than ever, or carry a chip on your shoulder? Have you developed a mistrust of friends? Do you feel trapped, doubtful of your ability, or chronically tired with no great physical activity to account for the tiredness?

Perhaps just a little personal stock-taking will ease the tensions. If your job is getting to you, changes may have to be made. But jobs aren't tense; people are. If a change is needed, it's probably you who will have to make that change, for you'd probably be just as tense in a new job.

If you feel overburdened with work, pitch into one task at a time. Get at the most urgent jobs and the others will no longer seem so overwhelming. Make certain you're not overburdening yourself with a compulsive urge to achieve perfection. Perfection isn't possible, and the effort to achieve it can be an invitation to failure.

Diversify your patterns; work, but then get away from the work. Physical activity, even no more than a brisk walk, can dissipate a lot of tension. When tension builds up inside, it dwells not just in the mind but in the whole body, including the muscles. Take a walk, or do anything else physical you feel like doing or can persuade yourself to do. Then come back to the problem.

Take a hard look at your treatment of and reactions to other people. If someone upsets you, try to figure out why. The upsets may come more from your own feelings than from anything the other guy has done.

A disagreeable boss or one who even seems personally hostile can produce intolerable tension on the job. Conceivably the hostility is personal, but the chances are that it isn't. Maybe he's more wound up and tense than you are. Maybe his wife isn't talking to him. Some things just have to be endured, and a disagreeable boss may be one of them. But nobody lives forever, and one way to win the battle is to outlive him.

When you're tense and worried, it often helps to talk your troubles over with a person you trust and consider levelheaded. Letting your problem out can relieve some tension, and your confidant may have some valid advice. Just airing your problem may give you a useful new perspective on it.

When your tensions and anxieties become too severe to be eased by such measures, your physician, if he's a good and interested one, may be able to provide some help himself. If he can't, he can refer you for psychiatric aid. That doesn't necessarily mean years on a couch; often a lot of good can be accomplished in half a dozen or fewer sessions.

How much influence on health does level of income have?

Considerable, as you might expect. And the influence shows up not only in terms of general health but also in terms of specific diseases.

Diabetes is one major disease that ranks among the top ten killers. It is also significant because it may contribute to deaths from other diseases, particularly heart disease.

A recent national survey of people with diabetes found a higher prevalence in families at lower-income levels. Families with incomes under $3,000 reported that one-third of their members had diabetes whereas in families with incomes of more than $10,000 one-eighth were afflicted with diabetes.

Insurance studies show generally higher death rates from diabetes among industrial policyholders (who tend to be poorer people) and lower death rates among standard policyholders. When a descriptive profile was drawn up recently for the woman who would have a high risk of developing cancer of the uterus, it depicted her as a woman of 30 or more years of age with low socioeconomic status.

At various times over the past fifteen years, the Medical Division of Du Pont has studied chronic disease among Du Pont employees, taking economic status into account. The studies show that income level is influential for many conditions. Du Pont employs 115,000 people, 85 percent of whom are male. About 60 percent are hourly paid production workers; the remainder are salaried in white-collar jobs. Employees range in age from seventeen to seventy-four. Those under forty are examined every two years by company physicians; after forty, they are examined yearly.

For the studies, employees were considered under five income classifications. Level I covered officials such as plant managers, district sales managers, research and laboratory directors, and office managers. Level II included attorneys, engineers, physicians, office supervisors, foremen, and accountants. Level III included salesmen, technicians, lab assistants, clerks, and bookkeepers. Level IV covered messengers, shipping clerks, draftsmen, and craftsmen. Level V included laborers and service workers.

For heart attacks, the incidence rates in the two highest categories were well below those in the lower-income categories. Over an eleven-year period, the incidence was 2.25 per 1,000 men in level I as against 3.99 in III, 3.57 in IV, and 3.16 in V. For strokes, too, the incidence was lowest in higher-income groups and progressively greater in lower-income groups. The rate in level V was twice that in level I. For high blood pressure the rate was lowest in higher-income groups, greatest in lower. More than twice as many men in level V were obese as in level I. For diabetes, prevalence rates were lowest in higher-income groups, and for cancer the men in level I had lower risk than the others.

Thus in all diseases studied the lowest rates were found consistently in the two highest-income groups and usually the rates were lower in level I than in level II.

The investigators suggest that the personalities, backgrounds, and living habits of men in higher levels may be sufficiently different from those in lower levels to account for differences in disease rates. Personal qualities required for managerial and executive positions, such as emotional stability and the capacity to cope with stressful situations, may also be related to protective mechanisms against disease.

The poor actually feel less healthy, don't they?

They do. A poll taken by Louis Harris and associates for Blue Cross Association found that one-third of American adults are concerned over not being able to sleep at night and about

one-fourth of those who smoke are upset over not being able
to stop. About 25 percent of people feel too exhausted to get up
in the morning and about the same number either lack appetite
or feel unable to control it. A majority, 52 percent, report being
lonely and depressed some of the time, and 23 percent said they
have felt emotionally disturbed.

And the poll found that poor people feel less healthy than
others do. For nearly two out of three ghetto blacks and poor
whites, "feeling fine" actually means "not as sick as usual."

When asked to compare the health of their own families with
that of times gone by, three-fourths of affluent Americans
answered unhesitatingly that health is better now. But among
the ghetto blacks and poor whites, the reaction was exactly the
opposite; most felt that they are sicker than the previous generation was.

According to the poll, 53 percent of the public has some
specific current ailment. Broken down into economic groups, the
figures are 44 percent for the affluent, 65 percent for inner-city
blacks, and 72 percent for Appalachian whites.

"As with serious illnesses and with minor afflictions," the
Harris report noted, "the poor lead everyone else in not feeling
right. The poverty groups . . . tend to be more 'worried and nervous,' more 'lonely and depressed,' less able to sleep, far more
exhausted, with less appetite, far more 'faint and weak,' and
more 'overly tense.' Only on the single item of 'can't control
appetite' are the poor less beset than the rest of American
people."

*What are the special problems of the poor concerning medical
care and health practices?*

There is a myth that the poor and the wealthy get the best of
medical care. "The truth," as Dr. George G. Reader of Cornell
Medical College has pointed out, "is that the poor commonly
receive inferior medical care, and despite government assistance,
it is likely to be expensive for them. Frequently they have to
choose between buying medicines, even at reduced rates, and
eating. This is a hard choice for both patients and physician,
but particularly for the patients. Lack of carfare may be crippling the search for medical care. We found in a study of welfare
clients that providing carfare was one of the most important
moves we could make.

"Another barrier to good health is lack of education. In a
number of studies we have found that clinic patients who have

not gone beyond the eighth grade in school do not understand modern principles of hygiene, or do not know about the diseases that afflict them. Accordingly, they fail to take the proper kind of precautions that the rest of us learn to take automatically. At first we thought the greater knowledge of those who had gone to high school was the result of health education courses. A more likely explanation is that if one gets beyond the eighth grade he is more inclined to read books, newspapers, and magazines, and so be exposed to sources of information."

Dr. Reader also notes: "Another problem for the deprived in the poverty culture is inability to comply with a medical regimen. The poor are not really accustomed to complying, for their survival often depends upon noncompliance. Furthermore, when a physician prescribes medicines for them to be taken at a regular hour, he may discover that they do not have regular hours. For instance, eating patterns among the poor are very irregular indeed. There is equal difficulty with other hygienic measures such as rest, sleep, and exercise. When the patient finds a regimen too complicated to follow, he often deceives the doctor by pretending that he is following instructions.

"Also in the poverty culture there is virtually an absence of preventive measures. The poor have little understanding of the importance of prevention, of knowing, for example, that an immunization this year may protect one next year. In many immunization campaigns, it was the poor who were least likely to appear for their injections."

One recent study adds to the evidence that insufficient personal care is an important mechanism affecting health among the poor, but it also provides a bit of encouragement. Investigators checked on a sample of 401 mothers with children aged nine to thirteen living in a northern New Jersey city. The families were from three socioeconomic levels. The top level consisted of families with total incomes of $10,000 or more and with husbands who were managers, owners, or professionals. The middle level ranged in income from $6,000 to $9,999, and the husbands worked in clerical, sales, skilled, or semiskilled occupations. The low level consisted of families with incomes under $6,000 and with husbands in unskilled jobs.

The differences in health practices in each level were particularly marked in certain areas such as exercise, nutrition, and dental hygiene. The lower the income level, the less likely the women were to exercise or engage in sports. Ninety percent of the low socioeconomic group, compared with 69 percent in the higher-income groups, engaged in no sports or games. Twenty percent of low-income women, compared with 10 percent of high income, failed to eat breakfast; 40 percent of low-income women, compared with 28 percent of high-income, failed to include all major food groups in the dinner meal. Seventeen percent of the poor, compared with 1 percent of higher-income women failed to brush teeth regularly.

More than 50 percent of the high-income group, compared with fewer than 30 percent of the low, had general checkups when not ill; 33 percent of the low, compared with 12 percent of the high, failed to see a physician within the first three months of pregnancy. The high-income group members were much more likely than the low to have had dental X-rays, cleaning of the teeth by a dentist, urinalysis, and smallpox and polio immunizations.

The higher the socioeconomic level, the greater the use of specialists such as dermatologists, orthopedists, optometrists, ophthalmologists, surgeons, and psychiatrists. The higher-income women scored significantly higher as a group on a test of health knowledge. Over half the low-income women were obese compared with 20 percent of those with high income. Twice as many low-income women had experienced indigestion or nausea within the past two weeks, both problems that can be associated with faulty nutrition and exercise patterns.

But the study found that people with a lower socioeconomic status who nevertheless maintained good health practices showed no disadvantage in level of health compared with those in higher socioeconomic groups. That is, when health practices were good, the level of health was equally high in all the socioeconomic groups.

Does marriage confer any health advantages?

Curiously, although many people believe that a single person generally tends to be more nervous, fearful, or psychologically distressed than a married person, recent findings do not support this belief. According to a government survey, people who have never been married show fewer signs of emotional disturbances at all ages than people who are married, divorced, separated, or widowed. They apparently suffer less nervousness, have less fear of nervous breakdown, feel less dizziness, and have fewer headaches and heart palpitations.

Despite this peace of mind, single people aren't favored when it comes to staying alive. The death rate for single men is more than double that of married men in the twenty-five-to-thirty-four age group, and the difference increases as men get older. For women of all ages, the mortality rate is almost twice as high for single women as for married women.

As one wag has put it, "Better wed than dead." But, according to another, "If married men live longer than single, it only seems longer."

How much unhappiness is there in marriage?

That's hard to measure accurately. One reflection of it, of course, is divorce. According to the U.S. Census Bureau, there were 47 divorced persons for every 1,000 married couples in the country in 1970, a 33 percent increase over 1960, when there were 35. It's also estimated that 600,000 couples separate each year, though not necessarily to get divorced.

Of every dozen marriages, according to studies by Dr. John F. Cuber of Ohio State University, four will end in divorce; six will be "utilitarian," with a few shared satisfactions to hold them together (such as children or career); and only two of the dozen will be what might be called "total" marriages, in which the couples enjoy doing everything together and enjoy sharing love that lasts a lifetime.

Curiously, polls show that nine out of ten men, if they had it to do all over again, would marry the same woman—but women don't return the compliment. Three out of four say they would not pick the same husband. Studies of dissatisfied wives produce two major complaints: husbands don't talk to them enough and don't live up to their social expectations.

What are the real anxieties and frustrations associated with marriage?

Somebody once called marriage "the incredible entanglement of two people." According to some experts, a common denominator in the breakdown of most marriages is the failure of one partner to meet the other's dependency needs. One or both partners may be seeking security and protection, a strong need that may stem not only from an unhappy childhood but also from a happy one. Failure of a spouse to fulfill the role of parental surrogate can produce emotional conflict and distress in the dependent partner. The conflict can be compounded by anger, which may lead to punishing behavior toward the mate followed by feelings of guilt and fear of retaliation. Such a relationship can become an emotional tangle, and sometimes a frustrated dependent spouse may use exaggerated illness as a weapon.

Some psychiatrists also point to marital one-upmanship. As one recent analysis put it: "The subtle force of competitiveness operates in many marriages to create a chasm between husband and wife. Not generally a direct cause of marital breakup, it nonetheless generates tension and hostility. In this area of conflict, both partners are dedicated to the game of one-upmanship. One investigator draws a parallel between it and the business ethic of profit and loss—neither partner is convinced of a 'gain' unless it inflicts loss upon the other. . . . A remarkable dramatization of vicious game-playing between husband and wife is Edward Albee's play *Who's Afraid of Virginia Woolf?* In this instance, the marriage did indeed endure—at least through act 3. So, in fact, do many in actual life which are based on pathologic needs. As has been observed, neurotic bonds of marriage are at times stronger than healthy ones."

Does business interfere significantly with marriage?

The *Wall Street Journal* is a business publication. And in a recent article it noted, "The corporation is taking the place of the Other Woman in the so-called eternal triangle—and the staggering impact on executive marriages suggests that big business is the most demanding mistress of all."

The article went on to note that even when a household is not upset by repeated geographic transfers, marriage may be affected because the company comes first in the husband's mind. If his energies are almost totally absorbed by his work, he may function inadequately as husband or father. And while divorce is not unduly common, particularly among junior executives, since it is bad for careers for young men on the way up, the marriage may become a mockery. Sex may be the first area affected; a resentful wife may punish her husband's frequent absences by refusing sexual relations. She may also take comfort in alcohol or promiscuity.

Obviously, all marital problems can't be blamed on "the office." A man who works to excess may be doing so not because the company demands it but because he has a drive to achieve. Or, conceivably, he may overwork because marital in-fighting makes him want to stay at work, which he finds more satisfying and less emotionally draining.

How common is infidelity?

According to some studies, 75 percent of all married men today have extramarital experiences, up from 50 percent in

Kinsey's day. Some investigators report that one-fourth of married women admit to having had some type of extramarital experience by middle age.

Infidelity may be more common today, but so, it appears, is increased tolerance. According to Pennsylvania State University sociologist Dr. Jesse Bernard, infidelity may still be grounds for divorce, but it is no longer reason for divorce. She found that only one-fourth of women confronted with an unfaithful husband would end the marriage.

Most psychiatrists would agree that in many cases infidelity is only a symptom; that fears about one's own sexuality can lead to experimentation with other partners, and depression and anxiety may be involved.

Some investigators observe that if marriage is regarded as an overall life partnership, the fidelity of the flesh becomes a small part of the picture. Often, if one partner has strayed from sexual fidelity, the other partner can be seen to have strayed from fidelity to the total marital relationship.

Not only don't extramarital affairs necessarily split a marriage; paradoxically, says one psychiatrist, they can have at least in a few cases a remarkable healing effect on the marriage. While infidelity disturbs the lives of both partners, each may become stronger for having come through the crisis. In some couples there is closer companionship and greater love life afterward.

Don't many people enjoy living alone?

A lot more *are* living alone, but they do not necessarily enjoy it. Latest census figures show a 43 percent increase in "single-person households" in the sixties. While the number of people in the fourteen-to-thirty-five age group has grown by 24 percent since 1962, the number of them who live alone has increased by 84 percent in the same period. In 1960 59.7 percent of nineteen-year-old women were single; in 1968, 70.4 percent were single.

People who live alone are concentrated in big cities. In the past five years, fifteen apartment buildings called South Bay Clubs have opened in Southern California. Only singles are admitted, and there are now 12,000 residents. On Manhattan's West Side, certain food stores cater to singles, selling milk by the pint, single lamb chops, and small cans of almost everything.

To some extent, changing moral attitudes have probably reduced the pressure to marry. With sex so free today, marriage isn't essential for that part of life. Yet many find drawbacks to the single life. As one single puts it: "For many people, living alone can be depressing. Married people have the fantasy that the lives of single people are all pleasure. When you're alone, there's no one to turn to, no one to support you, and no one to do anything for you."

Is there any help for the unhealthy marriage?

The modern approach is to consider that both partners are in need of therapy. Treatment for married couples may include successive therapy or analysis of husband and wife; concurrent therapy (simultaneous treatment by the same therapist but at different hours); conjoint therapy (simultaneous treatment of husband and wife in joint sessions); collaborative therapy, with two therapists, each seeing one partner; four-way sessions, with a different therapist for each partner and regular joint sessions in which all four meet; various types of group therapy; and family therapy, directed mainly toward the parental relationship.

Hopefully, therapy provides opportunity to learn different patterns of behavior to replace the patterns that caused distress. It is often pointed out that if two people learn to get along more positively in marriage, they may also increase their ability to derive emotional rewards from interactions with the rest of the world.

8

Personality

Are certain kinds of disease linked with certain types of personality?

Life is full of stresses. They're inevitable. In one sense, stresses can cause disease, but more strictly speaking, stresses are indirect causes. It's not so much the stress but the individual's personality and reaction to the stress that determines whether any harm is done.

Primitive medicine men may have had a point: They worked on the theory that psychological factors had much to do with disease. In recent years the germ theory of illness has grabbed the spotlight. But germs are always with us. You're full of germs right now; everybody is; but not everybody is sick. Something else must determine when germs make us sick.

Very likely behavior is a factor—even for germ-involved illnesses. Edward A. Suchman, sociology professor at the University of Pittsburgh, not long ago remarked: "Man today may be viewed as the 'agent' of his own diseases—his state of health is determined more by what he does to himself than what some outside germ or infectious agent does to him."

Because medical science now has control over many of the once-fatal germ diseases but we are still plagued with the chronic degenerative diseases, more and more medical men are looking to an "ecological" theory of disease. This theory, as Suchman says, considers disease to be a maladjustment to the physical and social environment and emphasizes the relationship of attitude and behavior to health. Increasingly the idea is that if we're going to have any further significant change in longevity, it's going to have to come through changing attitudes and behavior.

Dr. René Dubos has put it well: "Driving a car through heavy traffic, working at a frustrating job, watching a child struggle with illness, quarreling with one's mate—the stresses of life take infinitely varied forms. And they can pose just as much of a challenge to health as bacteria, viruses, malnutrition, or chemical and physical forces. Each man meets his challenge in his own way. The family quarrel that triggers a heart attack in one may only make another resentful, while for a third it may even serve as a goad to useful and productive work. Whatever the response, it involves the whole person; both body and mind play a part in dealing with the stresses of life."

But how could behavior and personality have anything to do with, say, cancer?

Consider the case of a midwestern farmwife, hard-working and phlegmatic. For twenty years she had cared for a mentally retarded daughter. When the daughter died, she took it stoically. A few months later, another daughter married against her parents' wishes and cut herself off from the family. A few months after that the woman, never sick in her life, collapsed and within a month was dead of cancer.

The woman had suffered two great losses and had refused to discuss them and discuss her emotions. Was her own death from cancer coincidental? It might have been dismissed as that if similar coincidences hadn't been discovered in the lives of hundreds of cancer patients studied. The studies increasingly support the concept that the way a person handles emotional stresses may somehow set the stage for the development of cancer.

One study in Scotland compared 200 lung-cancer patients with 200 patients without cancer. The cancer patients were found to be less emotionally reactive, without outlets for emotional release.

At the University of Rochester, a study of more than 100 patients with leukemia and lymphoma found that such cancers are likely to arise at a time when a person is reacting to a loss or separation with feelings of sadness, anxiety, helplessness, or hopelessness. A similar reaction has been found among patients with other forms of cancer.

Dr. Sydney G. Margolin of the University of Colorado has reported that the Sioux Indians, whom he describes as having few emotional inhibitions, are nearly totally free of cancer. And cross-cultural studies suggest that countries where cancer death rates are high also rank high in emotional inhibition.

Dr. Clauss Bahne Bahnson, professor of psychiatry at Jefferson Medical College, Philadelphia, argues that while emotions can't be said to cause cancer, they may set the stage for growth of cancer cells. "When a loss occurs, rather than going through a typical cathartic mourning process," he says, "these [cancer-prone] persons tend to deny the loss, adopt a Pollyanna attitude that says everything is fine, and keep on with their activities as if nothing had happened. Instead of their emotions being expressed in behavior, they go through the central nervous system which in turn affects the body hormones and immune responses in such a way as to permit the development of cancer."

Does sickness usually follow emotional upset?

Not always, of course. But at the University of Rochester a massive research program has been under way in psychosomatic medicine, the relationship between emotions and the body. Dr. George L. Engel and Dr. Arthur Schmale have found that the majority of patients hospitalized for a physical illness had a psychological disturbance shortly before they got sick.

The most common disturbance, they've found, is an attitude of helplessness, of giving up. "It was just too much," a patient would say, or, "I just couldn't take any more." The feeling of helplessness usually follows the loss or threatened loss of someone or something close to the patient—a spouse, parent, child, home, job, or planned career.

Thousands of such interviews at the University of Rochester Medical Center suggest that if a person responds to an event in his life with a sense of hopelessness, helplessness, or giving up, he may somehow initiate a biological change that fosters the development of an already-present disease potential.

Dr. Schmale and Dr. Howard P. Iker were able to predict the presence of cancer with 75 percent accuracy based on psychiatric interviews with fifty-one women who had entered the hospital for a cervical biopsy. The women all had had Pap smear tests indicating possible cancer of the cervix. Schmale and Iker predicted that eighteen who had responded to some recent situation in their lives with feelings of hopelessness would turn out to actually have cancer. Of these, eleven in fact did have it. Of thirty-three predicted to have no cancer, twenty-five did not have it.

Dr. Schmale explains these and other similar findings this

way: "Man is constantly interacting with his many environments, and at many levels of organization—from the subcellular and biochemical to the most external or peripheral, that of family, work, and now even his universe. We postulate that when a person gives up psychologically he is disrupting the continuity of his relatedness to himself and his many environments or levels of organization. In making such a break, or with this loss of continuity, he may become more vulnerable to the pathogenic influences in his external environments and/or he may become more cut off from his external environments and more predisposed to internal derangements. Thus, disease is more apt to appear at such time of disruptions and increased vulnerability."

Dr. Engel emphasizes that it is not the magnitude of an event but how a person reacts to it that determines whether he gives up. A seemingly minor event such as the loss of a pet may to some people be the last straw, whereas others would not give up even after loss of family, home, and job.

Is it always a matter of giving up?

Perhaps not a formal giving up, but an unhappy reaction to stress.

For example, in one study, 20 of the sickest and 20 of the healthiest among a group of 336 working women were compared. There were no significant differences in economic or cultural backgrounds, exposure to infection, or constitutional factors. But the sick women as a group thought of their childhoods as having placed great demands on them, they felt the same about their adult lives, and they found their lives unsatisfying.

Another study kept track of 3,000 people over a twenty-year period. Some stayed healthy. But some experienced repeated illnesses in certain years, and these people turned out to have certain characteristics in common. The cluster-illness people saw life as difficult and unsatisfactory. They reacted sharply to events, took things very seriously, tended to be anxious, self-absorbed, unduly sensitive. In contrast, the well group found their lives relatively satisfactory, and saw themselves as having good marriages and rewarding careers.

Are specific personality types prone to specific diseases?

Some work, particularly that of Dr. Franz Alexander and his colleagues at the Chicago Institute for Psychoanalysis, suggests so. For example, they see the typical rheumatoid arthritis sufferer as one who has difficulty handling hostile and aggressive feelings and tries to curb them, exercising great self-control but also a kind of benevolent tyranny over others. The arthritis may be set off when there is a loss of a person he or she dominated.

Asthmatics don't all fit into the same category, but in many cases, the Chicago research suggests, the asthmatic as a child inhibited his crying for fear of being rejected, particularly by his mother. He grows up with a frustrated desire to cry, which is sometimes manifested by a kind of frustration of breathing—asthma.

The person with high blood pressure often is one who swallows his hostilities, has trouble asserting himself, tends to be overly responsible, works hard and doggedly, feels increasing resentment, and lives in a state of tension.

The Chicago investigators are busily trying to sharpen such psychological profiles and draw them up for many kinds of illnesses, hoping they can be useful for physicians and perhaps even provide guides to avoiding the illnesses.

Personality seems to be very much involved with heart disease. Investigators have drawn up a relatively clear-cut personality and behavior picture of individuals most likely to have heart attacks. They virtually impose their own stress. But before we get to that, it's a good idea to get a look at just what stress is capable of doing.

How do you define stress?

You can call it the body's set of involuntary reactions to the demands of living. Better yet, instead of demands of living, say the dangers or seeming dangers that may arise in living.

Early man had to have these completely unthinking, instantaneous reactions to survive. They mustered his physical resources to meet threats. When he suddenly encountered a threatening beast, he had to fight or flee. If he were to do either successfully, he needed an extra surge of strength. Immediately his body accommodated. Into his blood poured extra amounts of hormones from his adrenal glands; his pulse, breathing, and blood pressure shot up; energy was mobilized from sugar and stored fats, and dispatched to his muscles and brain; and any digestive processes going on were turned off so they wouldn't use up energy.

Modern man has the same set of stress reactions, although it's rare today that he is presented with situations where he has to fight or flee. The same stress reactions, however, can be triggered by situations that make him fearful, anxious, frustrated. If he sees something as a threat to his job, if he reacts with frustration to a traffic tie-up, if he becomes provoked by spouse or child—out pour the adrenal hormones and the stress reactions are on. But there's no physical outlet for the extra energy; it's bottled up. And if he develops chronic patterns of stress, he pays a physical price.

What's the physical price of stress?

Under more or less continuous stress, some vital body part can give way, leading to a variety of illnesses and eventually to death.

Dr. Hans Selye, director of the Institute of Experimental Medicine and Surgery at the University of Montreal, developed the concept of harmful stress by exposing laboratory animals to many types of stressful conditions: extremes of temperature, loud noises, frustrating situations, such as being tied spread-eagled to a board.

No matter what the stress-provoker, if it had to be endured for long periods, it produced havoc in the body. Upon autopsy, experimental animals were found to have peptic ulcers, enlarged adrenal glands, and disturbances in other body glands.

There are three stages of stress, according to Selye. In the alarm stage, the body reacts to stress, whether it's a physical stress or an emotional one such as nervous tension. The alarm stage is followed by the resistance stage, in which the hormones keep pouring out and the energy is maintained at high level to deal with the stressful situation. But this is supercharged living, and if it's kept up for a prolonged period, the exhaustion stage sets in and one or more body organs are impaired.

Selye has pointed out that depending upon the stress agent's intensity and the individual's predisposition, a heart attack can occur at any point along this progression. His concept was first presented in 1950. Since then considerable evidence has been piling up that stress, especially emotional stress, plays an important part in coronary heart disease. It does so by elevating blood pressure and by increasing the heart rate, leading to increased work and strain for the heart. It also affects blood fats involved in clogging the coronary arteries feeding the heart.

Does stress raise cholesterol levels?

It does, as shown by many studies, both human and animal. Checks on students when they were preparing for final examinations and on income tax accountants under heavy pressure just before tax deadlines have shown higher cholesterol levels, than at other times. Air force men exposed to stress have shown higher levels than in nonstress periods.

When twenty navy underwater demolition trainees were repeatedly tested during their first two months of training, their cholesterol levels were up whenever they were angry, depressed, or fearful.

Because motor racing is full of emotional stress, a British researcher took blood samples from sixteen racing drivers both before and at various intervals until three hours after a race. The men were young (twenty-two to thirty-nine) and healthy. Hormone levels in their blood shot up a few minutes before the race, and dropped to normal fifteen minutes after. Fat levels in the blood also were high immediately before and immediately after the race.

At the University of Oklahoma, investigators worked with volunteers, keeping diet, exercise, and other factors constant, but subjecting some to emotional stress. There were marked cholesterol elevations in those undergoing stress.

A few years ago the Oklahoma researchers discovered the rather remarkable town of Roseto, Pennsylvania. They found that Roseto has an unusually low incidence of deaths from heart attacks, which is all the more intriguing in view of the eating habits and weights of the people. Of the 1,630 inhabitants, 95 percent are Italian. The town was settled in 1882 by immigrants from Roseto, Italy. Over a seven-year period, the investigators found no deaths at all from heart attacks in men or women under age forty-seven. And, overall, the death rate in Roseto from heart attacks was half that of Bangor, a town only a mile away. The same physicians and hospitals cared for the populations of both towns.

Rosetans work in small garment factories, nearby steel mills, and electrical industries. They eat a great deal and drink considerable amounts of alcohol, mainly in the form of wine. One of their favorite dishes is prosciutto, a pressed ham with a rim of fat an inch thick; Rosetans eat it whole, without discarding the fat. Cooking is usually done with lard. Rosetans dip bread in lard gravy. They apparently eat substantially more fat than the average American. And almost invariably men and women over age twenty-one are overweight. Their fat-eating and obesity should make them early candidates for heart attacks. Why the low death rate from heart attacks?

Apparently, the relative absence of stress saves the lives of the Rosetans. The striking feature of Roseto, the researchers noted, "was the way in which the people seemed to enjoy life. They were gay, boisterous, and unpretentious. The wealthy dressed and behaved in a way similar to their more impecunious neighbors. The visitor's impression of the community was of a one-class peasant-type society made up of simple, warm, and very hospitable people. They were found to be mutually trusting (there is no crime in Roseto) and mutually supporting. There is poverty, but no real want, since neighbors provide for the needy, especially the recent immigrants who still continue to arrive in small numbers from Italy."

After the first study, the investigators made a second for four more years. Over the entire eleven years, there were no deaths from heart attacks in Roseto among men and women under age forty-seven, in sharp contrast to neighboring communities.

Actually, Roseto inhabitants seem to have much in common with Benedictine monks, who live in rural areas, removed from the stresses of urban life, and in monastic environments free from economic problems. Monks of the order eat as much fat as other Europeans—and, as one American medical investigator notes, as much fat as the harassed general practitioner of medicine. But the monks suffer from coronary disease only about one-fifth as often as the doctors.

Does stress have any other ill effects?

Take a look at all the chief risk factors for coronary heart disease: high cholesterol levels, overweight, high blood pressure, lack of exercise, cigarette smoking, diabetes. Consider, then, suggests Dr. Henry I. Russek, that "it is well recognized that emotional tension may result in compulsive eating, drinking, and smoking in many persons as compensation for anxiety. Moreover, it does frequently contribute to the failure to achieve daily exercise by promoting fatigue, creating a sense of time urgency, and decreasing motivation. Nervous strain of occupational, cultural, social, or domestic origin is known to elevate blood pressure, to increase the tendency to obesity, to contribute to excessive smoking and lack of exercise, to participate in hypercholesterolemia [high cholesterol levels], and aggravate diabetes through psychic influences. . . . Even such indirect effects of emotional stress, barring all others, must elevate this factor to a position of considerable significance in coronary heart disease."

An interesting identical-twin study adds to the argument that stress is important in heart disease. Navy medics studied thirty-two pairs of identical male twins, forty-two to sixty-seven years old. One member of each pair had heart disease, the other did not, or one member of each pair had severe heart disease, and the other had mild. Both members of a pair, of course, shared the same inheritance—so that factor was out.

The investigators paid particular attention to four psychosocial factors: devotion to work, lack of leisure, home problems, and life dissatisfactions. These could be stress factors. The study found that men who had experienced heart attacks were far more devoted to work than the others; those with minimal or no heart disease showed the best ability to relax during their time away from work; those with more severe heart disease had a greater number of home problems, generally centering around economic arguments; and those with more severe heart disease were more dissatisfied with their lives.

Beyond those findings, another seems significant: of even more importance than work, leisure, and home-life patterns was how the subject *viewed* those and other areas of his life. The study suggests that an individual who works long hours, takes little leisure time, reports domestic strife, and all the while enjoys his life enormously may not be as vulnerable to heart disease as a person with similar life patterns who is largely dissatisfied.

This confirms what Dr. Stewart G. Wolf observed some years ago about the coronary-prone individual: that he is like the mythological Sisyphus, who passed the time in Hades pushing a large rock up a steep hill and never quite getting it there. The coronary disease candidate, Wolf argued, is a person who not only meets a challenge by putting out extra effort, but who takes little satisfaction from his accomplishments.

What overall behavior pattern is considered most unhealthful?

According to some of the most provocative of all recent research, a distinctive personality and behavior pattern seems to be characteristic of those people headed for coronary heart disease and heart attacks. This research was done by Dr. Meyer Friedman, a cardiologist, and his colleagues at Mount Zion Hospital and Medical Center in San Francisco. But psychiatrists in the past had noted clues to the role of personality in heart disease.

In the mid-thirties, Drs. Karl and William Menninger noted that many patients with coronary heart disease seemed to be aggressive, but only under the surface. A decade later, one psychiatrist wrote of a large group of coronary patients that they were hard-driving, single-directed personalities. Another described this group as aggressive, compulsive strivers who, although they tried to keep their aggressive impulses under control, justified to themselves a considerable amount of outwardly expressed hostility.

It wasn't until the mid-fifties that Friedman and another cardiologist, Ray H. Rosenman, began to establish an impressive case for the importance of personality and behavior in coronary heart disease. Friedman and Rosenman investigated the influence of such factors as cholesterol, smoking, blood pressure, and obesity in heart disease. They began to be impressed by the fact that their coronary patients had certain traits they saw less often in other patients. Out of curiosity, they sent a questionnaire to more than 100 business executives and also to 75 physicians treating heart patients.

The questionnaire included a list of possible causes of heart attack: smoking, lack of exercise, anxiety, obesity, and the rest. But it also included, as a possible cause, "excessive drive and meeting deadlines." The executives were asked to consider friends and acquaintances who had heart attacks and to check what they thought might be the main reason; the physicians were asked to do the same in terms of patients they had treated for heart attacks. It seemed significant that less than 10 percent of both groups, executives and doctors, believed that anxiety had anything to do with triggering a heart attack and 75 percent of both groups pointed to excessive drive and meeting deadlines.

Since then, Friedman and Rosenman have been building up their case for the existence of two major types of personality, A and B, with A being the coronary-prone behavior pattern. Most of us are mixtures of both types. But usually one or the other type is predominant and of course there are varying degrees of predominance.

How do you recognize an A person?

If anyone with behavior type A had to wear an emblem indicating his personality, it might well be a clenched fist holding a stopwatch, Friedman has suggested. The A person is aggressive, ambitious, and competitive; he has intense drive, has to get things done, and makes a habit of pitting himself against the clock.

Typically, an A person appears to be briskly self-confident. He is decisive in the way in which he speaks and even in how he moves and sits. He has a determined look, never dawdles, and even lights a cigarette briskly. His speech is rarely weak or monotonous; in fact, he tends to use various words of his sentences as "battering rams." He is often involved in many jobs, many civic activities. Friedman has observed that if a man has been told by his wife to slow down, chances are good he has type *A*.

Typically, too, an *A* person is aggressive and full of hostile feelings. If he plays games, even with his kids, he plays to win. He loves to compete with fellow workers. When it comes to his associates, he'd much rather have their respect than their affection. If anybody interferes with or delays what he wants to do, you can sense his hostility in his voice or even see it on his face.

But if any one thing most distinguishes an *A* person, it's time urgency. Almost never satisfied with his accomplishments, an *A* person is very much conscious of time and has a huge need to try to get more and more done in a given period. He is punctual to a fault, can't tolerate waiting even briefly for a table in a restaurant, can't tolerate having anyone take a long time to get to the point of a conversation and will often interrupt and try to speed the process.

Extreme *A* people can go to ridiculous lengths to get more things done. As Friedman has noted, "Some subjects like to evacuate their bowels, read the financial section of the newspaper, and shave with an electric razor, all at the same time. One subject admitted that he had already purchased ten different electric razors in his efforts to find one that would shave faster than all others, and another subject liked to use two electric razors at the same time so he could cut his shaving time in half."

What about pattern B *people? Are they dolts?*

Hardly. The *B* person may be just as serious, but he is much more easygoing, can enjoy leisure, and doesn't feel driven by time. The *B* person can be ambitious, but in a quiet, more reasonable way. He is easier to get along with, harder to anger. An *A* person usually has little or no respect for a *B*, but it is not unusual for a clever *B* to use an *A*. It has been said that while *A* people are more likely to be the top-notch salesmen, it is the *B* people who are more likely to be the corporation presidents.

Just how does pattern A *relate to heart disease?*

In one early test Friedman and his colleagues had one group of lay people pick from among their friends those who seemed to them to be typical type *A* people. They furnished eighty-three men. Another group was then asked to supply eighty-three men who seemed most typical of type *B*.

When all the men were thoroughly examined, twenty-three of

the eighty-three type *A* men (28 percent) had clear-cut symptoms or electrocardiographic signs of coronary heart disease. In contrast, only three type *B* men (4 percent) showed any evidence of heart disease.

That doesn't mean that generally any type *A* person will have seven times as much risk of coronary heart disease as a type *B* person. The eighty-three men in each category in the study were extremes. But the results did suggest that people with type *A* behavior are relatively prone to heart disease and those with type *B* much less so.

The same kind of study was carried out for women, with 125 type *A* and 132 type *B* women chosen by lay people. Most of the *A* women worked in industry or in professional jobs; most *B* women were housewives. The *A* women had more coronary heart disease (19 percent) than the *B* women (4 percent).

More evidence for the influence of type *A* behavior has been coming from a study that Friedman and his associates began in 1960 with support from the National Institutes of Health.

The earlier studies had picked men and women from the general population and found those with type *A* behavior were suffering from coronary heart disease four to seven times more frequently than those with *B*. But they didn't prove that *A* subjects *without* heart disease would develop the disease in the future more often than *B* subjects would.

The new study covered 3,500 men, age thirty-nine to fifty-nine, who had no indication of heart disease. They were examined, interviewed, and classified as type *A* or type *B*. Four years later, fifty-two had developed a first heart attack and eighteen had a first attack of angina pectoris indicating coronary heart disease. The incidence of the disease was three times greater among the type *A* than among the type *B* men. This study is still going on. At this writing, 257 of the men have developed coronary heart disease and 70 percent of the victims have been type *A*'s.

The researchers experimented to see if the behavior pattern— or some specific aspect of it, such as working under deadlines— might affect blood cholesterol. They got the help of a group of accountants who agreed to take blood tests twice monthly for six months. The accountants showed no particularly well-developed *A* or *B* patterns under normal circumstances. But when they were under special stress just before the April tax deadlines, their blood tests showed that their cholesterol levels were significantly higher than at other times. During the six months of blood testing, some of the men encountered personal stressful situations, which they reported to be more severe than tax-dead-line stresses. When blood cholesterol was checked at such times, it was markedly higher than at other times.

When cholesterol levels were checked in women, the levels in type *A* women proved to be considerably higher on the average than those in type *B* women.

It also appears that extreme type *A* men and women tend to smoke more cigarettes per day than *B*'s and also to find less time and have less inclination to exercise or engage in recreational physical activity.

What can A *people do to change the odds?*

It's no easy matter to change one's whole personality and be-havior pattern. But it would appear that anything an *A* person can do to relax a little, to stop constantly cramming more activi-ties into his life, could be helpful.

There's no avoiding stress. Extreme type *A* people complicate matters by themselves adding stress to their lives. But everybody faces stress, and it's not necessarily bad. Only protracted, un-relieved stress may cause trouble.

A few fortunate people can shrug off excessively stressful situ-ations. Anyone who can't and is faced with a continuously frus-trating job may find it wise to quit and get another; however much of a wrench the change of jobs may be, it's better than having to face a disabling or deadly illness.

Distraction can be good medicine for stress—reading, a movie, walking, almost anything that takes your mind off the stressful problem. In modern life most of the stress is mental and emo-tional, and physical activity is a particularly good distraction and escape valve. Says one physician: "Half an hour in the basement with a punching bag is a good way to relieve problems. And it's preferable to knock the hell out of a tennis ball than to take out your hostitlities and frustrations on your wife or secretary."

Dr. Paul Dudley White, the famed cardiologist, remarked: "To get physically tired is the best antidote for nervous tension. In my own case, nervous tension and strain can be counteracted, even prevented, by regular exercise."

What if one's daily routine is so hectic it leaves no chance for time out?

Schedule appointments with yourself before you get involved in more commitments. And be ruthless about it. Says one physician whose patients include many top-notch businessmen: "I insist they put limits on the time they donate to worthy causes. After a certain point, I tell them to give money instead. One may feel guilty about buying one's way out of obligations but these men, like everyone else, need some time off by themselves. And this is the only way they'll get it." Pick your own escape route, but be sure to schedule some diversion in your life.

In 1895, when Louis Pasteur was dying, he thought about his long scientific argument with Claude Bernard. Pasteur had shown that germs cause disease; he believed they were, in effect, all that mattered. On the other hand, Bernard had argued that germs were always present, all about, and were resisted by a person's "milieu interieur," his internal equilibrium; Bernard maintained that only when the equilibrium was upset, weakening the "terrain," did the germs take over.

On his deathbed, Pasteur finally agreed: "Bernard was right. The microbe is nothing, the terrain is everything."

9

Sex Life

Does sex have anything to do with longevity?

According to an ancient theory, asceticism is the father of longevity. Anchorites are supposed to have attained long life almost as a matter of course. Saint Simeon Stylites became a centenarian and, according to Saint Joseph, his main activity was holding himself "erect on a column forty cubits high in an attitude of continual prayer while undergoing an extraordinary fast." The anchorite Paul is believed to have lived to 113, contenting himself with "water, a few dates, and a bit of bread that Providence sent him every day."

There have always been those who advocate, if not total abstinence, at least major restraint in sexual activity as paving the way to long life. Throughout the history of modern man there has been debate about optimum frequency of intercourse for health, based on the idea that it's not wise to squander a given amount of capital energy that cannot be replaced.

No valid scientific evidence suggests that sexual activity leads to an early grave. Witness many octogenarians still very much active after a lifetime of anything but abstinence.

Actually, there's something to be said for the life-prolonging value of a good sex life, especially in view of all the so-called stresses of modern living. The sex act can be a matter of plain lust or an expression of love in the most intimate way. When sex is combined with love, something more than physical gratification may come of it. One discerning physician likes to think of

141

a good sex relationship in terms of the Greek myth of Antaeus, who was the son of the earth goddess. Whenever in combat Antaeus was hurled to the ground, he arose more powerful than before, for he drew strength from contact with his mother Gaea (earth).

The physician observes, "When a man and woman in love meet in the sexual embrace, each, like Antaeus, hopes to arise stronger than before, to go his individual way. In day-to-day living, the man who is diminished by a world that forces him to compromise or accept defeat finds total acceptance in the arms of the woman who loves him. And the woman who feels diminished by niggardly chores and obligations receives heartfelt homage from the man who loves and desires her. With sex and with love the man restores her integrity and she restores his. When the act of sex is truly an act of love it unites two committed human beings, obliterating their painful awareness of being alone and lonely. And the pleasure of the embrace, together with the certainty that tomorrow they will embrace again, gives them new strength to stand alone."

In other words, sex has considerable potential for easing tensions and stresses, for serving as a reinvigorating force.

But doesn't sex inevitably wane with age?

Not inevitably. Actually, older people *can* lead active sex lives but too often they're repressed by taboos and inhibitions. An idea that love and romance belong only to the young is most assuredly false.

At the Reproductive Biology Research Foundation in St. Louis, psychologist Alexander P. Runciman—a colleague of William H. Masters and Virginia E. Johnson, the authors of *Human Sexual Response*—studied the sex lives of 100 men and women ranging up to eighty-nine years of age. Some of the oldest in the group had plenty of active libido.

Runciman reports that when decreased sexual activity in older men and women occurs it is often related more to psychological than to physical factors. Many persons continue to lead active sex lives in their seventies and eighties. Others are physically able to have sex, but use the alibis of "advanced years" and "inadequacy" as respectable excuses for ending sex.

Can lack of sex lead to disease?

It may induce prostatitis in men. No reliable figures exist, but it has been estimated that as many as one-third of all men, commonly younger men in their twenties and thirties, suffer from prostatitis.

The prostate is a gland that adds a secretion to semen at the time of ejaculation. The secretion appears to potentiate the activity of the sperm in the semen. Prostatitis is an inflammation of the prostate, which can produce a chronic feeling of discomfort and pain in the perineum, the external area between testicles and anus. Repeated sexual stimulation without satisfaction is a cause of the inflammation. Regular sexual intercourse is a cure. And if regular intercourse for any reason isn't possible, regular masturbation is a help.

Isn't sex supposed to be bad for the heart?

Supposed to be, yes. There have been a lot of stories of men dying of heart attacks during intercourse.

In fact, there have been quite a few quasi-scientific anecdotes on the subject. And, as a recent editorial in the *Journal of the American Medical Association* pointed out, many physicians caring for patients recovering from heart attacks prohibit coitus for some time after such episodes. This ban seems reasonable, since the heart rate speeds up during the sex act. But, the editorial asks, what's the evidence that a heart attack may occur or recur? And it answers that in all the medical literature there is only a single report of death from a heart attack apparently suffered during intercourse. "And this report is so brief and poorly documented as to be only slightly more reliable than the average, and probably apocryphal, newspaper account of similar 'events.' . . . Perhaps, considering current trends to promote physical exercise in postinfarction [after heart attack] patients, we should prescribe sexual intercourse for those individuals as therapy."

Does sexual activity relate in any way to cancer?

A study of more than 31,000 nuns in the United States shows that they are much less likely than other women to develop cancer of the cervix. On the other hand, they are more likely than the average woman to develop cancer of the breast, the uterus, the ovaries, and—somewhat surprisingly—the colon.

Many still unanswered questions are raised by the study. But some current thinking runs this way: Cancers of breast, uterus, and ovaries may well be influenced by the level of female sex hormones. Increased production of these hormones during pregnancy may well be the reason why women who have borne children have lower risk of breast and genital cancer. Conceivably, that reasoning may also apply to cancer of the colon, which takes the lives of more than 18,000 American women annually, more than any other form of cancer in women except breast cancer.

If further research supports the finding that childless women are more likely than others to develop colon cancer, that evidence at least would be helpful from the standpoint of giving such women the benefits of regular checks to detect the disease in early stages. Possibly, too, as some cancer experts have suggested, oral contraceptives, which create a hormone environment similar to that of pregnancy, might have some useful protective effect against breast, genital, and colon cancer in childless women.

Can cancer be transmitted from one partner to the other during intercourse?

The idea that cancer is contagious—that a man, for example, can contract penile cancer from his wife's uterine cancer or vice versa—is *not* valid, but the myth persists.

If cancer were contagious, nurses, doctors, and surgeons, all of whom come into contact with cancer without using any special precautions, would have a frequency of cancer higher than that of the general population—but they don't. And cancer does not spread through the family of a cancer patient.

Cancer transmission from one individual to another has not been seen in humans. Perhaps the closest case is that of cervical cancer. The normal uterus is shaped like and roughly the size of a pear. The elongated lower part, which opens into the vagina, is the cervix. Cancer of the cervix is the most common of uterine malignancies.

A tremendous amount of data on cervical cancer has been collected. Prostitutes have been found to have six times the cervical cancer rate of the general female population. The disease is virtually unknown in nuns and virgins. It is less common in women married once than in those married several times. It occurs most frequently in women who began sexual intercourse in their teens. It is more frequent in women who have intercourse with many partners. It occurs less often when condoms are used by the male partners.

It appears that circumcision of males has an effect on the risk of cervical cancer of their sex partners. The lowest incidence is among Jewish women. Jewish males are circumcised soon after birth. The cervical cancer incidence also is low among Moslem women, whose husbands are circumcised. It is lower in circumcision-practicing African tribes than in other tribes. And cancer of the penis is very rare among men circumcised early in life.

The foreskin, or prepuce, of the penis has under it a secretory gland that produces a fatty substance called smegma. Circumcision, which removes the foreskin, permits smegma to be washed away without difficulty. In the uncircumcised male smegma accumulated under the foreskin may be deposited in the vagina during intercourse.

Smegma has been implicated in cancer of the penis. While many investigators feel that at this point it can't be assumed to be directly responsible for all cervical cancer, smegma appears to be at least a promoting agent capable of inducing cervical cancer in association with some still-unknown agent.

Circumcision, then, is a good health precaution?

Most doctors would say that circumcision has great hygienic value; a minority call circumcision a "mutilation" seldom justified for medical reasons. According to that minority, soap-and-water hygiene is just as good.

Common in the United States (an estimated 60 to 90 percent of all male infants are routinely circumcised), the operation is universal among Jews and Moslems. It is rarely performed in most European countries, China, and some other Far Eastern areas.

Aside from possible preventative value against penile and cervical cancer, many physicians believe that circumcision helps prevent other conditions. One is phimosis, in which the foreskin is too tight to be retracted. Another is balanitis, inflammation of the head of the penis. These conditions are not uncommon in Sweden for example, where circumcision is not routine.

It has been suggested that circumcision diminishes sexual pleasure. The theory is that removal of the foreskin exposes the penis to constant contact with clothing and thus dulls its sensitivity. Experiments conducted by Masters and Johnson of the Reproductive Biology Research Foundation found no significant differences in penile sensitivity of circumcised and uncircumcised men.

Is there an ideal frequency for intercourse?

No. Appetites vary. Statistics totted up by various investigators suggest that the overall average may run about twice a week, more often for the young and the newly married, less for others.

Many factors are involved: opportunity, sexual compatibility, temperament, and presence or absence of fatigue. Whatever the frequency, if both partners enjoy intercourse and are relaxed afterward, it's probably a good frequency.

Is potency reduced by frequent intercourse?

Intercourse doesn't decrease potency and abstention doesn't increase virility. Sexual relations several times a day may, indeed, decrease the amount of sperm a man produces in each ejaculation. But even then he doesn't exhaust his potency. There may come a point where he needs a rest; chances are he'll want it because of satiation rather than potency exhaustion.

Are women relatively undersexed?

Far from it. Until very recently in modern times, society insisted that women be sexually pure before marriage. After maintaining chastity before marriage, many women experienced some sexual self-consciousness after marriage, finding it difficult to make the transition. But the potential is there. "The sexual potential of a woman is not less but far greater," observes Virginia Johnson, "for unlike a man she can immediately go on to another orgasmic experience."

Does organ size affect sexual satisfaction?

Rarely, if ever. But it's commonplace for men to worry about penis size and for women to worry about having too large a vagina to give pleasure or too small a vagina to allow intercourse without pain.

Actually, it's a matter of technique. Even if a penis is markedly undersized or a vagina markedly enlarged, there are ways of going about the sex act that produce plenty of satisfaction. It's a fact, too, that with sexual excitement, the vagina can enlarge sufficiently to accommodate even a very large penis.

Is there any truth at all in the idea that masturbation in youth is harmful?

Masturbation is *never* physically damaging. Some psychic problems, however, could stem from unjustified fears and guilts associated with masturbation.

But the harmfulness idea hangs on. It may be indicative that an otherwise intelligent college student wrote a letter recently to a physician who conducts a weekly medical question-and-answer column for the campus daily: "I write this letter out of frustration from masturbation. Can masturbation cause hair loss?" The physician's reply: "I receive a large number of questions concerning harmful effects resulting from masturbation, but I'm still waiting for a testimonial to the beneficial effects."

Indeed, there may be beneficial effects of masturbation. Today many medical men go beyond the placid reassurance that "it won't hurt you if you are moderate about it."

Dr. Philip M. Sarrel of the Yale University Medical School, joining with Dr. H. R. Coplin of Amherst's psychology department, recently wrote in the *American Journal of Public Health*: "Concerning self-stimulation, we disagree with the injunction that 'it won't hurt you if you don't do it too much'—what is too much?—and affirm that for some individuals, women included, it can enhance the development of sexual response; under some conditions it can serve as a substitute for coitus, can temporarily relieve honest sexual tensions, and need not result in self-devaluation."

Masters has pointed out that many married men and women masturbate on occasion, for good reason and with no harm done. The reasons may include sickness, separation, or just plain impulse. He says, "Many women will masturbate with the onset of their menstrual cycle if they are having dysmenorrhea—severe cramps. An orgasmic experience frequently will relieve the spasm of the uterus and the cramps will disappear. Many women learn this trick. Does it work for all? Of course not, but it helps some women and so they masturbate, which seems sensible."

Masturbation is a very common practice. As far back as the Kinsey studies, 92 percent of all men interviewed said they masturbated at some time; 88 percent of unmarried men age twelve to twenty admitted practicing it. And some 50 percent at age fifty said they masturbated. The practice among women is no less common.

What about the dangers of abnormal sex practices?

What's abnormal? Insertion of penis into vagina is normal. But is there really anything abnormal about any other sexual practice that provides pleasure?

Actually, concepts of normal and abnormal depend largely on society's value judgments. Increasingly now, as the result of a change from the highly moralistic approach of previous generations, what once were considered abnormal practices, or perversions, are being thought of as deviations and before too long they may be classified simply as variations.

Dr. Judd Marmor of the University of California Department of Psychiatry points out that in the first millennium of the Christian Era virginity was not prized, marriage was a temporary arrangement, and extramarital affairs were taken for granted in many parts of Europe. Incest was frequent. Women aggressively invited sexual intercourse. Bastardy was a distinction; it implied that some important person may have slept with one's mother.

Marmor also notes that in feudal times, it was the feudal lord's prerogative to deflower any bride and in some societies all the wedding guests copulated with the bride. Such practices were considered ways of actually helping marriage, because any pain of initial coitus couldn't be associated in the bride's mind with her husband.

"It was not," says Marmor, "until the medieval church was able to strengthen and extend its control over the peoples of Europe that guilt about sexuality began to be a cardinal feature of Western life. Even the early Hebraic laws against adultery had nothing to do with fidelity but were primarily concerned with protecting the property rights of another man (the wife being considered property). Married men were free to maintain concubines or, if they preferred, multiple wives; also there was no ban in the Old Testament on premarital sex. The medieval church, however, exalted celibacy and virginity. . . . At one time it went so far as to make sexual intercourse between married couples illegal on Sundays, Wednesdays, and Fridays, as well as for forty days before Easter and forty days before Christmas. (By contrast, Mohammedan law considered it grounds for divorce if intercourse did not take place at least once a week.)"

Is sex really an instinct, a driving force,
that has to be satisfied?

That's an important question that concerns many people— people who worry because they don't seem to be as interested in, and driven by, sex as others. They think there must be something inherently wrong with them. But there may be nothing at all wrong with them.

Biological factors definitely influence sexual behavior. But the terms long applied to sex—"urge," "need," "impulse"—suggest that it is *all* a matter of a driving force. These terms were applied long before there was any modern research into human sexual behavior.

Among the indications coming from such research is that sexual behavior in humans, while it may have an instinctive base, may also be very much of an acquired taste and habit, considerably dependent upon learning experiences in the course of growing up. This experience factor could account for wide differences in sexual behavior among people.

Talking to a British audience recently, Derek Wright, lecturer in psychology at the University of Leicester, pointed out, "If sexual desire is learned and cultivated, then obviously there is no biological standard of sexual behavior against which to assess ourselves. Norms in this matter are completely social. If we want to ignore them, we can. The sexologists have sought to liberate us in the area of our sexual relationships. Now, to my way of thinking, liberation in sex means being able to take it or leave it. The biological-energy idea claims that it's impossible to leave it, but when we recognize that it is to a large extent learned, we begin to realize that it is also a matter of choice whether we have it or not."

What causes impotence?

The possibilities are almost endless, in theory. Impotence—the inability to have an erection—can stem from a wide variety of causes, both physical and mental.

Congenital defects, endocrine gland disorders, nervous system or urogential injuries can cause impotence. Prostatitis can produce impotence. So may diabetes. Chronic debilitating illness of any kind, major surgery, serious accidents, or a heart attack may produce some degree of impotence. Extreme fatigue, mental or physical, can cause temporary impotence.

A large amount of alcohol may reduce potency. Heavy drinkers often have some degree of impotence, and there's evidence that much hidden alcoholism is to be found in men who complain of impotence, although doctors often miss it.

Some barbiturates and tranquilizers may produce impotence as a side effect. Impotence often occurs among heroin addicts. Some investigators even report that some degree of sexual difficulty often *precedes* heroin addiction.

But the major factors in impotence are psychological. Anxiety probably plays a significant role in every case of impotence. Even when a man has a chronic physical illness, it may be the emotional repercussions more than the illness itself that affect sexual performance. Anxiety may also stem from work stresses, adjustments to a new job, promotion, loss of job, demotion, any frustrating life experience, and—quite commonly—any sign of sexual difficulty or feeling of inadequacy. As one physician put it, the simple thought "How am I going to make out this time?" can be fatal to erection.

It's the rare man who occasionally doesn't experience an episode of impotence. The cause may be just plain fatigue, or preoccupation with a business problem, or a bit of excessive drinking. If he fails to understand the reasons for the first episode of impotence and assumes that something is wrong, excess worry may set off a "fear of failure" cycle, which can lead to chronic impotence. Some men develop a "fear of failure" cycle based on concern about the myth that virility must inevitably be lost with age.

It should also be noted that some men discover that when they marry the woman with whom they've had successful premarital relations, something goes wrong and they develop some degree of impotence. A psychiatric explanation offered for this situation is that to some men there are "good" and "bad" women; when a "bad" woman becomes, as a wife, a "good" one, she is suddenly forbidden as a sex partner. Some men, to be potent with their wives, have to think of them as prostitutes.

Is impotence treatable?

Of course. Therapy can be as simple as brief counseling on drugs or dinking. It may be a matter of treating a health problem, such as diabetes. When the problem is psychological, sometimes simple reassurance is enough, and psychiatric treatment—not necessarily long, drawn-out analysis—often helps.

What is frigidity?

Frigidity means many things to many people. Literally, it means total unresponsiveness to the sex act, and that condition is extremely rare. But the term is also applied to everything from repulsion by and avoidance of sex relations through lack of orgasm to orgasm achieved only part of the time.

Women sometimes use sex as a marital weapon, giving or withholding as a means of controlling the marital relationship. Such women aren't necessarily frigid.

As with impotence, the causes of frigidity are infinitely varied; everything from inadequate stimulation or even insufficient lubrication to such problems as infection or inflammation of the clitoris, cervix, ovaries, or other organs.

But by far the most common causes are psychological. One physician tells of a young woman who after a few months of what had started out to be a happy marriage complained about a sudden loss of sexual response. She had no fault to find with her husband's sexual techniques, which are often responsible. Finally the physician asked what happened before sex—what happened from the time both she and her husband arrived home from work. It turned out that the husband usually began to make love right after dinner.

The physician, knowing the girl's mother to be a compulsive housekeeper, could make a guess about what might be wrong with the bride: while making love she kept thinking about the dinner dishes. Thanks to her mother's training, she couldn't leave them overnight in the sink.

"I solved the problem," the physician says, "by telling her to just go out and buy a large plastic dishpan and leave the dishes soaking in it in soapy water overnight. By morning, all she had to do was drain and rinse. That may hardly sound like a serious medical solution—but it worked."

Many psychological factors are capable of producing some degree of frigidity—lack of privacy, concern about finances, or other everyday problems. Old habits of thinking and feeling may be involved; a woman brought up in a sexually repressed atmosphere often is inhibited in sex because of the intrusion of old prohibitions.

What hope is there for the frigid woman?

Plenty. If there are physical problems, they usually can be overcome. Old habits of thinking and feeling may not be easy to change but they are not impossible to change. Sometimes, psychiatric help may be needed.

Can sexual worry produce physical illness?

That's quite possible. Consider a case, not unusual, reported by a physician at the University of Oklahoma Medical Center. A young wife visited at least a dozen doctors in an increasingly frantic effort to find a cure for her dysuria (severe pain upon urinating). Finally she found a urologist who examined her thoroughly and could find nothing physically wrong to explain the problem.

Quietly, he began to ask questions about her sex life. For the first time, she poured out a story of a husband more sophisticated at sex play than she was, or her upbringing permitted her to be. When he aroused her with oral-genital caresses, she allowed them and responded. But next day she suffered acute feelings of shame, fear, and guilt. In a matter-of-fact manner, the urologist assured her there was nothing at all wrong in her husband's acts; in fact, they were normal. In a few weeks, the young wife's dysuria was gone.

Is it worthwhile to seek help for sexual problems?

Today sexual counseling can have remarkable effects. Until very recently, most physicians were total losses when it came to the sex area, however competent they were in other departments. They had no training and they emerged from medical school with the same misconceptions and anxiety they may have begun with. As recently as 1966, only three medical schools in the United States had formal courses in sex education. But an increasing number of medical schools are now training their students in sex matters, and many physicians are going back for graduate courses.

If you have a sexual problem talk to your family doctor; if he can't help, he may be able to recommend a physician who can. Among specialists, gynecologists have shown considerable concern about sexual matters.

If you still can't find a physician able to help, you can write to the chairman of the department of psychiatry at the medical school nearest your home, stating your problem as frankly as you possibly can, and asking him to whom you should turn. Since he is basically a teacher, the chairman will rarely help you himself, but he can suggest someone who can help.

Is venereal disease on the rise?

For some years now, public health authorities have been warning that VD is getting out of control and that if something isn't done about it, it would cripple, incapacitate, and eventually kill more people than died in the Vietnamese war. Gonorrhea incidence has been hitting all-time peaks, with an estimated 2.3 million cases treated annually. Syphilis, which had been declining steadily in incidence, is on the increase, with more than 80,000 cases a year now being treated.

But the number of cases treated is no real indication of the true incidence of either disease. It's estimated that more than

500,000 people in this country are victims of undetected syphilis and in urgent need of medical attention. And as gonorrhea has increased, so has the number of women who act as unknowing reservoirs.

What are the symptoms of gonorrhea?

First of all, it doesn't always produce warning symptoms especially in women. Typically, in a man, there's a whitish discharge from the penis, with or without burning during urination, beginning three to seven days after exposure. Usually it's so uncomfortable to have an erection that there's no delay in seeking medical help. Gonorrhea can be knocked out with prompt and suitable antibiotic treatment. But it's been found recently that as many as 12 percent of infected men don't have immediate warning symptoms.

In women, while there may be a whitish vaginal discharge and some burning on urination, such symptoms often are not attributed to gonorrhea. Moreover, very often they are quite mild and even entirely absent.

What happens when gonorrhea is untreated?

In men, in some cases, the infection may eventually affect the prostate or the epididymis (a structure located alongside the testicle), causing severe pain and infertility.

In women, the infection may affect the fallopian tubes leading from ovaries to uterus, sometimes with spillover into the abdominal cavity, causing fever, severe abdominal pain, and peritonitis. Symptoms may be so severe that emergency surgery may be performed in order to make certain that appendicitis is not the cause.

Generally, antibiotics are effective against gonorrhea, and the outlook is good. But in some cases, particularly in those with repeated infection, even after adequate treatment there may be scar formation at the infection site. In men such scarring narrows the urethra and may obstruct urine flow; if it does, repeated dilation of the urethra or even surgery may be required to prevent scar tissue from closing the channel completely.

Women run a higher risk of infertility from repeated episodes of gonorrhea because the fallopian tubes may become chronically infected and scarred, and eggs from the ovaries then cannot pass down normally to the uterus. Abscesses may also form internally, requiring surgical drainage.

As many as 85 percent of women will show no immediate

symptoms of gonorrhea, and they can spread the disease unknowingly. Often the disease is not discovered in a woman until it is found in a man who has contracted it from her.

Does the Pill have anything to do with gonorrhea?

Aside from any role it may have in encouraging promiscuity, the Pill differs from mechanical devices and vaginal foams and jellies in that it presents no barrier to gonococcus, the bacterium that causes the disease. Some public health officials are urging doctors to emphasize to women that contraceptive pills will not in any way prevent VD. Says one official: "The indifference to pregnancy that the Pill engenders has carried over to an indifference to the possibility of other risks."

Another trouble with the Pill, some investigators report, is that it creates an alkaline environment in the vagina that encourages growth of the gonococcus. Older types of contraceptives, such as the diaphragm and jelly, foams, and powders, produced an acid environment that provides some measure of protection against infection.

What happens if syphilis is untreated?

Syphilis can be deadly if untreated. It has taken the lives of 3 million babies and 1 million adults in this country since 1900. In that period 100 million people throughout the world died of syphilis. The disease does its deadly work over a period of many years, and its early manifestations are so mild that they often are disregarded.

Syphilis can be transmitted to others only during the first two years after it is acquired. The first symptom is a sore, usually on the genitals, three to six weeks after contact with an infected individual. The sore will disappear on its own, but if the disease goes untreated the next symptom takes the form of a rash anywhere on the body and occasionally fever and sore throat. Once again, even without treatment, these symptoms disappear. But, if untreated, the spiral-shaped syphilis organism, *Treponema pallidum*, goes underground for years. Quietly, progressively, it attacks various organs without giving away its presence (except by a blood test). Finally, when damage has been done to vital organs, the patient seeks treatment. At this point, treatment can stop further damage, but it cannot completely undo the damage already done.

The great physician, Sir William Osler, once observed, "To

know syphilis is to know medicine." That is because the disease can affect virtually every organ. It can attack the brain and spinal cord, producing insanity, stroke, shooting pains throughout the body, or joint deformities. It can affect arteries and produce congestive heart failure or even heart attack.

Who gets VD most frequently?

There once was a flip but generally valid answer: the three Ps—the poor, the prostitutes, and the promiscuous.

No more. Today people of all walks of life may have venereal diseases. "Study after study," says a public health physician, "indicates that 5 to 10 percent of young women have gonorrhea, even pregnant young women, even pretty young women from nice families—even married women with grown children."

Another reports, "Even pillars of society, just returning from conventions and business trips, present themselves in increasing numbers each year in doctors' offices. Their harried and secretive attitude reveals their problem. The visit ends with a 'never again' promise—until the next year."

The upsurge in VD is worldwide. "Genital pollution," it's called by Dr. Thorstein Guthe, chief medical officer for venereal disease of the World Health Organization.

Modern travel is implicated as one cause of increased VD. People do a lot of roaming these days. One example: a prostitute's customer sought treatment for syphilis at the Sacramento County Health Department in Northern California. The woman was located and because she kept a diary of her customers showing the "home bases" of 310 of them—all sex partners during the time she could have spread the infection—a vast hunt began. Many of the men were located and treated. There were 50 from Texas, 25 from California, 20 from Arizona, 16 from Tennessee, 15 from Alabama, 13 each from Arkansas and Oklahoma, 12 from Minnesota, and 10 each from Florida and Missouri. There were others from each of the other states and 1 each from Canada and Mexico.

Don't doctors routinely report VD cases?

They are legally required to do so, and it would help track down VD carriers if they did. But physicians are often reluctant to do this. Some public health authorities say that doctors are especially reluctant when the victim is a prominent citizen or an old friend. One recent national survey found that although private physicians treat about 80 percent of the cases of VD that are treated, they report only one in nine to public health officials.

Are preventive techniques being developed?

An ideal solution would be a contraceptive that is also anti-venereal. Investigators are working on this, testing vaginal anti-septics and contraceptive jellies and foams in experimental animals. Some of the preparations show interesting possibilities, but the work is in very early stages. The best means of prevention available today is the condom.

Many authorities think that washing the genitals after sexual contact might well make a considerable impact in reducing risk of VD. The mechanical action of washing would reduce some germs; many others might be killed by the soapy fluid.

Actually, VD is not 100 percent infectious. On the average, for every five persons having intercourse with someone having syphilis, only one is likely to be infected; for gonorrhea, the figure is one in three. This suggests the likelihood that infection risk might be reduced further by washing. In World War II, when there was no penicillin, soap-and-water washing among the troops apparently did provide substantial protection. And some physicians think that washing may be an important reason for the relatively low gonorrhea rate in France, where the bidet is used.

10

Weight

Is a fat person doomed to a shorter-than-normal life?

Of course, other problems can shorten life. But statistically the overweight person, other things being equal, can expect to live fewer years than the person of normal weight. Suppose we could eliminate all premature deaths from cancer; that would add two years to the human life-span in this country. But if all deaths related to obesity were removed, the life-span would jump by seven years.

According to insurance figures, among overweight men the mortality from all causes is 150 percent of that for other men; among overweight women, 147 percent of that for other women.

Insurance statistics relate excess mortality to the amount of excess weight. For example, as compared with people who are somewhat below average weight, men who are overweight 10 percent or more have an excess mortality of one-third; for those overweight by 20 percent or more, the excess is nearly one-half. For women, excess mortality relates more precisely to the percentage of overweight so that those 20 percent overweight have 20 percent excess mortality and those 30 percent over have 30 percent excess mortality.

Does overweight increase the impact of specific diseases?

Compared with the population in general, overweight men and women have these excesses of mortality: 142 percent and 175 percent, respectively, from heart attacks; 159 percent and 162 percent from cerebral hemorrhage (stroke); 191 percent and 212 percent from chronic nephritis (kidney disease); 168 percent and 211 percent from liver and gallbladder cancer; 383 and 372 percent from diabetes; 249 percent and 147 percent from cirrhosis of the liver; 154 percent and 141 percent from hernia and intestinal obstruction. These insurance figures have been known for some time. More recently, an American Cancer Society study of 800,000 people found that obese individuals have one and a half to three and a half times as many fatal heart attacks and strokes as persons of normal weight.

Obese people also tend to have breathing difficulties, since the greater weight on the chest wall causes greater work in breathing. Because of their breathing difficulty, the obese have less tolerance for exercise. They have a higher rate of respiratory infection.

The obese frequently have impaired carbohydrate tolerance that may be sufficient to be classified as diabetes. Difficulties during anesthesia and surgery are associated with excess weight. In women with significant obesity, menstrual abnormalities and abnormal hair growth occur with some frequency.

It is well established by now that in treating many health problems, weight loss often is of considerable value. Among such conditions are high blood pressure, angina pectoris, congestive heart failure, varicose veins, spinal disk rupture, osteoarthritis, and many other varieties of bone and joint disease.

In 1959 a study by the Society of Actuaries revealed that thirty pounds of excess weight cuts four years off life expectancy. This statistic has been used by many insurance companies. Although policies are issued to the obese, premium rates rise proportionately with the amount of excess weight. These companies will cut premium rates when these policy holders reduce weights to accepted normal levels.

Exactly what effect does obesity have on heart disease?

Once it was thought overweight was a direct cause of heart disease. During World War II studies, particularly in Finland and the Netherlands where food often was short, showed that as caloric intake went down so did atherosclerosis (hardening of the coronary arteries leading to heart disease). So some people assumed that too much food produced the disease.

Today we know that many factors are involved in atherosclerosis and there are interactions between those factors. High blood pressure contributes to atherosclerosis. And obesity contributes to high blood pressure: a fall in pressure occurs in many obese people when they lose weight.

There's also that substance of ill repute—cholesterol. Cholesterol is deposited on artery walls during the process of atherosclerosis, and cholesterol in the blood increases during periods of weight gain. There's evidence that physical inactivity favors high blood cholesterol and, of course, inactivity favors weight gain.

Does obesity have only an indirect effect on heart disease?

No. But for a time even the Framingham study seemed to support that idea. That study, begun in the early fifties, has followed more than 5,000 men and women in Framingham, Massachusetts, and helped to point up many of the factors involved in coronary heart disease. It showed, for example, that cigarette smokers get coronary heart disease at many times the rate of nonsmokers; that a systolic blood pressure of 180 can double the expected coronary disease rate and that a cholesterol level of 260 or higher can do the same. At first the Framingham study and others as well seemed to indicate that if obesity existed by itself, unaccompanied by high blood pressure or high cholesterol levels, it did not (unless it was extreme obesity) increase the risk of coronary heart disease. But if obesity was present along with either high blood pressure or high cholesterol level or both, it did greatly increase the risk of a fatal coronary attack.

More recently the Framingham study has turned up some additional findings. In men the weight before age twenty-five and the weight gain after that age are strongly correlated with the risk of angina pectoris and sudden death, but not with producing a heart attack. In other words, obese men, whether or not they have elevated blood pressure and high blood cholesterol, have increased risk of angina pectoris and sudden death, indicating that obesity by itself contributes to these manifestations of heart disease. Basically, the study shows that obesity is dangerous when it adds to the work of a heart that already has some impairment of coronary circulation.

At one recent medical meeting, there were two interesting reports. According to one, heart attack runs in families, but if family members lose excess weight, their risk of heart attack is markedly reduced. At the Clinical Research Center at the Massachusetts Institute of Technology, Dr. Robert S. Lees and other researchers induced a group of moderately obese people (7 to 18 percent overweight) to reduce at the rate of one to two pounds a week. All had inherited a predisposition to excess blood fats. As they approached their ideal weights, their blood-fat levels fell to normal or near-normal. As a bonus, weight reduction often brought about a decline in blood sugar, blood pressure, and uric acid, all of which, in excess, also jack up the coronary risk.

It has long been known that the fatter you are, the higher your blood cholesterol level is likely to be. Now there's evidence that fatty tissue makes its own cholesterol.

At the University of Toronto, investigators bathed slices of fat tissue in solutions containing radioactively tagged chemical building blocks of cholesterol. They found the fatty tissue to be an adept cholesterol producer.

Then they compared the rate at which fatty tissue made cholesterol with the rate at which the liver made cholesterol (the liver has long been known to be the major manufacturer of cholesterol). Expressed in terms of production per unit of organ weight, fatty tissue turned out cholesterol at about one-fifth the rate of the liver. But since total fatty tissue in the body even normally is about five times the amount of liver tissue, the results suggest the volume manufactured to be about the same.

Unlike the liver, however, which slows down cholesterol production when cholesterol is eaten, the fatty tissue goes right on producing it.

Just how extensive is the obesity problem?

Nobody knows exactly how many people are carrying around too much blubber. Estimates run from 20 to 25 percent of all Americans. Preliminary results of a national nutrition survey, the first large-scale one, suggest that 25 percent is closer to the mark.

Weight gain used to be largely a phenomenon of middle age. By middle age the kids were grown up and life was a bit more tranquil and it was easier then to put on extra pounds. But today, in terms of body weight, many people are middle-aged by age twenty-nine; by then, they weigh as much as their forebears did in their middle and late forties.

Why is obesity so common now?

"Wealth is the parent of luxury and indolence," according to Plato. More recently, a New York health-club owner put it less articulately but pungently: "Layin' down and watchin' television after a meal, that's a mistake. In the olden days, they didn't do those things."

Our ancestors had to do rigorous physical work. A typical farmer in the past burned up 1,500 more calories a day than today's typical desk worker does. Grandmother burned up some 1,000 more calories a day than today's housewife with her modern laborsaving devices.

A clerk in 1900 got up at dawn, split wood and shoveled coal for the stoves, walked a mile or more to his job, walked home again, split more wood and shoveled more coal. He was considered to be a sedentary worker because his clerking job was sedentary. "In America today," Dr. Jean Mayer of Harvard has observed, "a physically active man is one who thinks he will play golf next Saturday. And a very active man is one who did play golf last Saturday."

Sedentary living, though, is not the whole story. Change in diet—a greater change than many of us realize—has had important consequences.

Not too many years ago there was no regular home refrigeration except for blocks of ice; food storage was limited; meat could not be kept in large quantities without spoilage, even in winter. Many families placed far greater dependence on vegetables and cereals than they do now. Fresh fruits and vegetables were eaten in quantity in summer and canned for winter use. The home-canned fruits contained no heavy syrup. More poultry was eaten, and beef, veal, and pork were raised differently and were leaner than modern livestock.

With refrigeration, mass production, supermarkets, and a rise in affluence, we have groaning tables. We eat more meat (from fatter animals) and are accustomed to many rich desserts. Most of us no longer eat just for survival. We have family meals, plus business and club luncheons, coffee breaks, and candy counters and snack and drink vending machines in office buildings and movie houses. Life today is full of opportunities for calorie consumption and, at the same time, has fewer opportunities for calorie expenditure. It's almost as if the system is against us, and we have to hunt ways to outsmart it.

Could there be something wrong with our
appetite-regulating system?

Our appetite-regulating system doesn't fit in with modern conditions because it evolved at a time when the chief threat to man's survival was lack of food, when long periods of starvation or semistarvation were experienced by almost every individual.

The appetite-regulating mechanism, Dr. Lawrence E. Hinkle, Jr., of Cornell University Medical College points out, generally causes an insistent hunger drive. It goes to work even within a few hours after a good meal, and the person driven by the mechanism goes looking for food again. At the same time, the satiation mechanism is weaker than the appetite mechanism; a person confronted with plenty of food can eat much more than he immediately needs.

Our appetite-controller had excellent survival value, in early hunting and fishing or food-gathering societies and even in primitive agricultural societies when a consistent food supply couldn't be counted upon.

But in this country, with our present food production and distribution techniques, food is always abundant. We don't need an insistent appetite to goad us into food gathering. We need a stronger satiation device!

When living in a setting where food is abundant, says Hinkle, "men have to make almost a conscious effort to avoid becoming obese. As a result of this, not isolated men, but whole populations have become relatively overweight, and have relatively high levels of fat and cholesterol in their blood. This is thought to be a primary reason for the high level of coronary heart disease in such societies."

Aren't there psychological causes for obesity?

According to some experts, people overeat for psychological reasons—to fill voids in their lives. They use food as a substitute for love or an escape from frustration. One psychiatrist tells of a patient who was impotent. "Whenever he had a strong sexual urge, he didn't go to bed with his wife. He raided the refrigerator."

According to one expert, people who are obese don't have a specific kind of psychological illness; they suffer the whole spectrum of such illnesses. But another retorts: "What's psychological or psychogenic? If we mean that not having the strength to rcsist food is psychogenic, then all obesity is psychogenic."

Is heredity involved?

Studies show that fewer than 10 percent of children of normal-weight parents are fat. The percentage goes to 50 percent when one parent is fat and to 80 percent when both parents are fat. But the question is whether this relationship results from genetic factors or from habitual overeating because of the way the family eats.

Some investigators point out that it's the rare mother who can stand to see a child with an empty mouth. Many of us, they argue, are the victims of our parents' memory of deprivation.

At Rockefeller University recently, investigators have discovered that fat people have three times more fat cells and that the cells are about one-third larger than those of people with normal weight. It seems that the excess could be related to infant feeding patterns. The Rockefeller scientists found that newborn rats that had to compete with only three other rats for mother's milk became much fatter than those competing with twenty-one other rats. After the baby rats were weaned and allowed to eat what they wanted, the weight differences remained. The fat rats had far more and larger adipose cells than thin rats.

And that, translated to humans, conceivably could mean that a fat infancy makes it tough to keep at desirable weight; the fat cells, the extra ones, don't go away.

Do fat people have a basically different eating mechanism?

At Columbia University, psychologist Stanley Schacter has found what looks like a basic difference in eating habits. Normal-weight people, he reports, are internally cued eaters; they eat when they feel hungry and feel hungry only when their stomachs are empty. No matter how much they may like a particular food, they are not tempted if their stomachs are full. If they become emotionally disturbed, their food consumption tends to go down.

On the other hand, Schacter finds that fat people are stimulated to eat by external cues *unrelated to hunger*—for example, the smell or sight of food, surroundings, time of day, emotions. They may have just eaten, but they can't walk past a bakery without being tempted. When upset, angry, or frustrated, they make an immediate trip to the refrigerator.

What kind of metabolic problems can lead to obesity?

Apparently, even eating too much at a meal may change metabolism and make a person hungry. Dr. Donald W. Thomas of Harvard has reported that oversize meals can alter the metabolism so that a large portion of the food eaten is turned into stored fat instead of available nutrients. As a result, finding itself deficient in *available* nutrients, the body sends out signals to start eating sooner.

The very fact of being overweight disturbs the body's metabolism, according to studies by Dr. Neil Solomon at Johns Hopkins

University Hospital in Baltimore. His work suggests that only 10 percent of people start out with a metabolic problem that can cause obesity. Others start out with normal metabolism and, by overeating, create metabolic problems.

The body produces more than 100 enzymes along with many hormones that affect metabolism. If any of these substances are not being produced in the proper amount, the process may be disturbed. For example, Solomon's work indicates that many overweight people may have a lower-than-normal amount of a liver enzyme. This enzyme produces a substance called crotonyl coenzyme A. Without this substance, fat may tend to accumulate in the body instead of being used up.

How can metabolic problems be corrected?

Solomon believes that most metabolic disorders don't require medication. Given a low-calorie diet—but a balanced one containing all the food elements needed for good nutrition—the body can usually restore its own metabolic balance. Fad diets won't do any good, Solomon insists, as do other authorities. If a metabolic disorder is involved, that's all the more reason to avoid freak diets that may further impair metabolism. Sound diets prescribed by a doctor may help correct the existing disorder.

How can anyone tell whether he or she is carrying around too much weight?

One way, of course, is to consult a weight table. Pick the right one and you can get some idea, but not necessarily a foolproof idea.

For many years, the standard table indicated weights for each year of age from fifteen up for men and women of various heights. But the weights were average ones based on those of some 200,000 people accepted for life insurance many years ago. The table was open to criticism. For one thing, the 200,000 people didn't necessarily represent the whole population. Also, the table showed a steady increase of weight with age, which probably isn't desirable.

Newer tables get rid of age as a criterion; in effect, they acknowledge that it's not good for average people to add weight with years. They also introduce the concept of desirable rather than average weight, a considerable difference because calculation of average weight includes the obese people who compose the upper part of the average.

But weight tables are not foolproof. If you find your weight is far above what the table says it should be, undoubtedly you are fat. But it's possible for someone to exceed his desirable weight and still not have any excess fat on him; that's true, for example, for some college athletes. On the other hand, it's also possible for some people to have excess fat without being markedly overweight according to a table; that's true for some very sedentary people.

To get a more direct measure of actual fat on the body, there are some simple tests. Simplest of all is just to stand naked in front of a full-length mirror and take a look at yourself. If you look fat, you probably are.

Another test involves just lying flat on your back and putting a ruler on your abdomen, along the body midriff. Usually, if there is no excess fat, the abdominal surface between the front of the pelvis and the flare of the ribs will be flat, so the ruler should lie flat. If it points upward at the midsection, you're probably toting some excess fat.

Another simple test for men is to compare the chest measurement at the level of the nipples with the abdominal measurement at the level of the navel. If the abdominal is greater, it usually means excessive abdominal fat.

There's also the pinch test. Just grasp skin between your thumb and forefinger at your waist, stomach, upper arm, calf, and buttocks. Most body fat is directly under the skin. Generally the layer under the skin—which is what you grasp since only fat, not muscle, pinches—should be one-quarter to one-half inch. With a pinch, you get a double thickness, so allow one-half to one inch. Anything above one inch indicates too much fat.

Do people normally get somewhat more lardy with age?

Yes, muscle tissue tends to be replaced to some extent by fat as the years pass, even if the same weight is maintained. Compare men in their twenties with older men in their late forties and fifties who have identical heights and weights. The older men have half again as much fat content in their bodies as the younger men do. It's much the same for women. People who keep physically active don't have as great an increase in fat content with age, but they have some.

If you have gained weight with age, you should make it a

point to stop adding any more excess pounds. Later, if at all possible, lose some weight slowly.

How successful are people in losing weight?

Not very. According to polls, at least three-fourths of over-weight Americans have made some try, however half-hearted, at controlling their weight. At any one time in this country 20 million people are on diets. Not without reason, dieting has been called the number one national pastime. It appears that the average dieter goes on 1.25 diets a year. And most studies show that the chronic dieter lucky enough to lose some weight promptly gains it all back.

Most dieting, unfortunately, is foolish and faddish. There are plenty of entrepreneurs around selling weapons to combat fat, weapons that have no more effect than popguns. Diet quackery is a $100-million-a-year business.

Where the next "magic" diet is going to come from is hard to say. There are wonder diets that concentrate on a single food, such as all eggs or all anything else. Other wonder diets use food pairs, everything from spinach and eggs to bananas and skim milk. The idea seems to be to melt off fat quickly during a short period of misery. But such crash diets have been known to produce acute malnutrition and even fatalities.

Every so often, a high-fat, low-carbohydrate or even no-carbohydrate diet turns up under a different name. With some alcohol added, the same kind of diet becomes a "drinking man's diet." Periodically, low-protein, low-fat diets come into vogue.

What's wrong with fad diets?

Even if they're not dangerous for lack of essential nutritional elements, they're self-defeating. Initial quick weight loss may be largely water loss rather than reduction of body fat. Even when real fat is lost, the dieter may well fail because the restricted diets are not acceptable for any extended period of time and he quickly regains weight returning to his customary eating habits.

It could very well be that people who use crash diets might be better off not dieting at all and keeping their excess pounds; at least they would avoid the risks of on-again, off-again weight fluctuation. Some evidence indicates that continual gains and losses may have bad effects. Blood cholesterol levels have been found to increase during periods of weight gain, increasing the likelihood that cholesterol will be laid down on artery walls. But there's no indication that, once deposited, cholesterol can be removed by weight reduction. Therefore it is possible that a person who repeatedly gains and loses weight may be subjecting his arteries to more fat-choking stress than the person who maintains a steady amount of excess weight.

A few words should be said here about skipping meals. On the surface, it looks like a smart idea. The trouble is that meal-skippers often nibble or eat too much at the following meal and end up taking in more total calories than they would have consumed in three normal meals.

Is there a sound approach to weight reduction?

Excess weight is usually a chronic problem. If a sudden bulge appears after a spree of overindulgence, maybe a crash diet can help. But the bulge that enlarges gradually over months and years is a matter that requires different handling.

One pound of fat in the body is the equivalent of 3,500 calories. To eliminate the pound, you need a deficit of 3,500 calories—that much more outgo than intake. A helpful guide is the 15× rule. If you're moderately active, it takes about 15 calories daily per pound of body weight to maintain your present weight. If you weigh 160 pounds, 2,400 calories a day will maintain that weight. If your intake is greater and your caloric expenditure—the number of calories burned up by physical activity—stays the same, you will gain. If you take in 100 extra calories a day, you're going to gain a pound in thirty-five days.

It also works the other way: Take in 100 calories less a day, and in thirty-five days you will lose a pound. You can lose weight by cutting down caloric intake, or by being a little more physically active or by a combination of the two. The 160-pounder, who needs 2,400 calories a day to stay at 160 pounds, can lose a pound in thirty-five days by any of several ways. He can consume 100 calories less a day. Or he can burn up 100 more (for example by walking an extra twenty minutes a day). Or he can use a combination, such as taking in 50 calories less and burning up 50 calories more by walking an extra ten minutes a day.

Most overweight people, of course, want to lose more quickly. They are conditioned to the idea of quick loss by all the fad diets. They want to start a diet, often a new one each time, and go through a short period of misery and be finished. The quicker the results, the better. Quick weight loss, however, may not be the wisest approach to weight reduction.

Does it hurt to lose too much too fast?

Dr. Sheldon Margen, chairman of the Department of Nutritional Sciences at the University of California at Berkeley, has done thorough metabolic studies that indicate that a loss of half a pound per day may be the maximum possible for losing fat alone without concomitant loss of muscle and other tissues.

He points out that one pound of fat equals 3,500 calories. To lose a pound a day, all of it fat, you would need a calorie deficit of 3,500 calories a day. But that's impossible because the average person burns up only 2,200 to 2,500 calories a day. The additional weight loss must come from protein tissue and water (for every gram of protein burned up, five grams of water are lost). Protein loss represents a danger signal to the body. Once you go off the quick-loss diet, the body will strive to regain the lost protein as quickly as possible.

Unless there is some special circumstance and a knowledgeable physician recommends greater loss, probably a pound a week should be tops. Even a loss of just half a pound a week adds up to a considerable loss—twenty-six pounds—in a year.

Aside from the extreme of trying to lose weight so fast that you lose vital protein, the ability to keep weight off still depends upon caloric balance between intake and output. The only successful diet will be one that takes pounds off at a reasonable rate and is itself so basically satisfying and appealing that you can live with it at a maintenance level.

In other words, having taken off weight, you should be able to go on eating in much the same way as you did during your diet, with a little more intake since you no longer need to have a caloric deficit.

A sound dieting program should do more than just take off pounds; it should teach you healthful eating habits. The new habits will allow you to avoid the yo-yo effect of frequent weight fluctuation and the potential ill consequences that accompany it.

Good eating habits can't be developed with severely restricted crash diets. You need a balanced diet with all the nutritional goodies—proteins, carbohydrates, fats of the right kind, vitamins, and minerals. By adjusting the balanced intake in terms of calories, you can get rid of excess poundage and at the same time continue eating a healthful, satisfyingly varied diet.

Are calorie tables necessary for good dieting?

It's possible to reduce simply by eating a little less, without religiously figuring out calorie counts. That's all the more possible if, at the same time, you engage in a little more physical activity than you've been accustomed to.

But many people find calorie counting helpful as a guard against overeating. It may seem tedious at first but the dieter soon learns the caloric values for his favorite foods, and the figuring becomes almost automatic.

What should the balance be between fats and other foods?

Considering what is known about fats and coronary heart disease, many authorities believe that a good diet should contain at least 14 percent protein, at most 30 percent fat (with saturated fats reduced), and the rest carbohydrates (with sugar cut to a low level). Those proportions, especially if a variety of foods is used, provide every essential nutrient; avoid excessively high fat intake, which promotes high blood fat levels; and avoid excessively low carbohydrate content, which may lead to fatigue and irritability. And you have enough fat and protein to promote satiety, a feeling of having eaten well and of being satisfied.

Just what happens during the process of losing weight?

According to Dr. Grant Gwinup, excess food calories are stored in the form of globules of fat inside millions of special cells, called connective tissue cells, most of which are located just under the skin. Normally the cells are small, shaped much like footballs. As fat pours into them, they swell and become just about as chubby as beach balls. When the body needs to use some of the stored fat, nerve signals go to all the fat cells and each pours out a tiny amount of fat through tiny blood vessels into the general circulation. When the body need is fulfilled, the nerve signals stop.

What exercises are best for burning up fat?

Gwinup observes that the more vigorous the exercise, the more fat it's going to consume. Burning excess fat involves combustion, which requires oxygen. Everything else being equal, the more an activity makes you huff and puff, the better for burning off of fat. But few people can go cross-country skiing every day, or play tennis for an hour a day, or take a fast swim every day. Practically speaking, you have to pick an activity that is convenient and doesn't become a burden. You might take a brisk walk, do calisthenics in your room, jog—anything that will make you breathe a bit hard.

Do commercially-produced low-calorie foods have any value?

Yes, but beware. Some so-called low-calorie foods actually contain no significantly reduced number of calories. Some people get a false sense of security out of low-calorie labels, tending to regard them as meaning calorie-free. Not uncommonly, a person may eat twice as much of a low-calorie product as he would of the normal food, but the low-calorie product may contain only 25 percent fewer calories. And some dietetic foods may have lower sodium content but not lower calorie content.

Do drugs help?

Many drugs have been used or promoted for treating obesity, but all have limitations. Thyroid extract is effective and safe only for people with hypothyroidism—underfunctioning of the thyroid gland. Only a fraction of the obese population has hypothyroidism.

Appetite-reducing agents—amphetamines and the like—depress appetite usually for only a few weeks, and in many people tolerance develops rapidly. If a person keeps increasing the dose because of tolerance (because starting amounts no longer work) toxic effects may follow. In individual cases, some physicians feel that an appetite-reducing agent may be of some use as a temporary aid, but no more.

Diuretic drugs—agents that promote loss of body water—are sometimes used in the early weeks of weight reduction when there is a discouraging plateau or leveling off of weight. Except for this brief period, few physicians believe their use is justified.

What causes weight plateaus?

These are brief periods in which there is no apparent weight loss even though the individual is eating no more and exercising no less. Such a plateau may occur at about the third week of dieting. Usually it involves a kind of rebalancing of the body after the considerable amount of fluid loss in the first week or two. Often the early fluid loss occurs because of a decrease in salt intake, as salt tends to hold fluids in the body. The third-week plateau is followed by further weight loss if the dieter continues to diet. There may be other plateaus because of increased salt intake and water retention. In time weight loss starts again as the body adjusts, if the diet is adhered to.

Does joining a diet club do any good?

It may; for many people the clubs are helpful in providing motivation. They vary greatly in their programs, but most emphasize planned diets coupled with lectures and experience sharing. Some prescribe particular exercises.

A diet club may require an initial medical certificate for membership, but few have continuing medical supervision. Some physicians say that because of the lack of medical supervision in some clubs, the condition of their heart and diabetic patients has worsened as a result of diet advice given. If you're thinking about joining a diet club, your doctor may have advice about which may be most suitable for you.

Are there drastic treatments for obesity?

Yes—starvation or surgery. One or the other may be necessary in a relatively few cases of life-threatening obesity or where obesity is involved in making diabetes unmanageable.

Total starvation or extremely low caloric intake (under 900 calories a day) should be an in-hospital procedure. It may cause abnormal heart rhythms, low blood pressure, and acute gouty arthritis. A close medical watch is needed.

Surgery essentially involves setting up new intestinal connections so food passes through less of the nutrient-absorbing small intestine. It can lead to various imbalances, and the surgery may have to be undone after several years, with subsequent return of obesity.

How can people of normal weight best maintain that weight?

One physician, who heads an organization concerned with executive health, has a philosophy that undoubtedly applies for all kinds of people. He advocates eating what you like and, no less important, liking lots of different things. That way, he says, you don't even have to analyze your meals to make sure they are balanced and giving you every nutrient you need.

He also suggests that it's a good idea to read a calorie table once or twice to fix in your mind the inordinately high calorie contents of foods like heavy desserts, snacks, fried foods, and alcoholic beverages. Then when you get the first indication your weight is starting up, it takes only a slight change in your eating habits—maybe just cutting out desserts for a while—to hold the line.

11

Physical
Activity

We hear much talk about the need for physical activity. Is there any connection between exercise and longevity?

The evidence keeps getting stronger that there is. Lacking fancy laboratory tests, many physicians, as far back as the early Greeks, have suspected that exercise has a general bearing on health. Recently evidence of specific values has been piling up. And there are insights into the how's and why's.

Nobody claims exercise is some kind of panacea. Obviously, exercise is not the only important factor for health and longevity. But it's important—and in many ways.

In what ways?

For keeping one feeling fit, and to some extent slowing the physical deterioration that begins for most of us in the early twenties.

As a help in combating many diseases and, it would appear, as a help in preventing some. For example, exercise may be a preventive and even a therapeutic weapon against heart disease. Not only is lack of physical activity a risk factor for coronary heart disease but also many of the other risk factors respond favorably to exercise. The factors favorably affected include even high cholesterol levels in the blood and high blood pressure.

What evidence is there of the relationship between exercise and a healthy heart?

In one of the early investigations in England Dr. J. N. Morris found that the frequency of coronary heart disease was about 30 percent less in bus conductors than in the bus drivers. The drivers sat all day; the conductors clambered up and down the double-decker buses. To Morris, the difference in activity level seemed to explain the difference in heart disease incidence.

Morris then conducted a national autopsy survey covering hospitals in Scotland, England, and Wales. He obtained additional evidence to support the theory that men in physically active work have less coronary heart disease than those in more sedentary jobs. He studied some 5,000 autopsy reports and considered the job activities of each subject. It turned out that physically active men—postmen, laborers, and others—not only had less coronary heart disease than sedentary workers such as schoolteachers but also the disease they had was less severe and developed later. Hearts of sedentary men showed damage equal to that of heavy workers ten to fifteen years older.

Similar studies have been done in the United States with similar results. For example, among 120,000 railroad employees, the incidence of heart attacks proved to be almost twice as great among office workers as among men working in the yards. A study of 2,000 District of Columbia postal workers showed that clerks had at least 1.4 times the risk of coronary heart disease as carriers.

Of more than 300 Harvard football lettermen followed up over a long period, 34 developed coronary heart disease. But no man who had kept physically active since leaving college had the disease.

One study of 3,263 longshoremen continued for sixteen years, during which 291 men died of coronary heart disease. The death rate for those with less vigorous jobs on the docks was one-third higher than for the others.

What does physical activity actually do?

One thing exercise does is to affect blood cholesterol levels. High levels of cholesterol are associated with clogging of the coronary arteries. If cholesterol is high, exercise can help bring it down and even help keep it from going too high in the first place.

In a famed Boston–Ireland study, Harvard investigators checked on 700 Boston residents of Irish descent and then compared them with their brothers who had stayed in Ireland. The men were in the thirty-to-sixty age range. The coronary heart disease death rate for the men in Boston was twice that for the men in Ireland. The men in Ireland ate on the average 400 more calories a day than the Boston men, but they weighed 10 percent less. Moreover, the men in Ireland ate more eggs, more butter, more other foods likely to elevate blood cholesterol levels, yet they had lower cholesterol levels. Why? More exercise, regularly, day in and day out for the men in Ireland. Beyond burning off calories, the exercise evidently kept cholesterol levels low.

Other studies show the same cholesterol-controlling effect. For example, 100 marines in rigorous training were fed upward of 4,500 calories a day, including plenty of saturated fat. At the end of six months of heavy eating but also of continuous hard work, the fat content of their blood was unchanged.

In Finland it has been found that lumberjacks eating a diet containing 44.7 percent of calories from fat actually have lower cholesterol levels than sedentary men who get 34.3 percent of their calories from fat.

In a trial at Kent State University in Ohio, forty-two men in sedentary jobs, age twenty-nine to sixty-three, volunteered to take part in a physical fitness program in which they worked out an hour a day, five days a week, for nine months. In every man, cholesterol level declined; the higher the level at the beginning, the greater the drop.

What are other specific effects of activity?

Physical activity may serve to ease tension. Anybody who has ever found himself, in the midst of stewing with anxiety or frustration, in almost violent need of getting up and moving around, has some idea of the ability of physical activity to relax the mind and body.

It's pretty difficult to stay all wound up with job or other worries and concerns while you're playing a game of tennis, or bowling, or jogging, or batting a ball with the kids.

Remember the stress concept: When anxiety occurs the adrenal glands pour out hormones to get you ready to fight or flee. You're mobilized for physical action. The energy has to go somewhere—and it's better for it to be used up by the muscles rather than have it add to turmoil within.

There is evidence that when the stress reaction isn't allowed a physical outlet, there is a bad effect on the arteries. The adrenal gland outpourings, in mobilizing the body for action, bring fats out of body stores to serve for energy. If they're not used for that purpose they float around in the blood and some may be deposited on artery walls.

Does exercise have any effect on high blood pressure?

There have been studies in which hypertension patients have exercised under careful medical supervision. For example, twenty-five hypertensive men took part in a study at the San Diego State College exercise laboratory. Their mean blood pressure was 159/105. After six months of a program in which they did warm-up calisthenics for fifteen to twenty minutes, then about half an hour of walking and jogging twice a week, the mean pressure for the group was down to 146/93.

It seems that a reasonable exercise program may have some value in curbing hypertension. There are indications, too, that exercise, insofar as it helps to keep weight under control, helps prevent hypertension. Hypertension is very much linked with excess weight; in fact, weight reduction is frequently used as treatment for elevated pressure.

What is the relationship between exercise and nourishment for the heart muscle?

A lot of blood moves through the heart chambers—all told, 2,000 gallons a day. But the heart gets no nourishment from this flow. What happens is this: As the heart pumps out fresh blood for the whole body, it goes first into the aorta, the great trunk-line artery that is about as big in diameter as a garden hose. From the aorta many arteries branch off to feed various areas of the body. And from the aorta branch off the two coronary arteries that feed the heart. The coronaries break up into smaller and smaller branches in order to get blood to every part of the heart muscle.

The whole system is very flexible and adaptable. Remember that many arteries branch off from the aorta to carry fresh blood to all parts of the body. The coronary arteries will take so much of the blood when you're at rest; they will take somewhat more when you're active and, because of your activity, the heart beats faster. The system is adaptable to serve your needs.

It can be adaptable another way. The more physically active you are and therefore the more active the heart, the more likely it is that coronary circulation system will be stimulated to increase collateral circulation, the formation of new branch vessels and connections that distribute blood to the heart muscle by another route.

The more extensive the collateral circulation, the less danger there is if a heart attack occurs. In a heart attack, a coronary vessel, increasingly narrowed by fatty deposits on its internal wall, shuts off completely so blood can't get through. As a result, part of the heart muscle is starved and it dies. That is the heart attack.

But if collateral circulation exists, it may be able to carry the blood right around the blocked portion—enough, in fact, so that the heart attack may not occur. If a heart attack does occur, the collateral circulation may help minimize it—actually reduce the amount of heart muscle affected.

Collateral circulation also may be the reason why some people, despite severe atherosclerosis—heavy deposits almost choking a main coronary vessel or even more than one—don't suffer from angina. Angina is the excruciating chest pain that usually takes place when a person who has severe atherosclerosis exerts himself. This is in effect the heart muscle's cry that it is not getting enough blood to support the increased heart work called for by the exertion. But if the person has led a physically active life, collateral formation may have been stimulated even as the atherosclerotic process was going on. In effect, the new collaterals will counterbalance the atherosclerosis. While less blood reaches the heart through the diseased vessels, that loss is made up by the blood reaching the heart through the collaterals. When that is the case, there may be no angina.

Investigators working with animals have been able to demonstrate the collateral formation. They've taken animals with some artery narrowing, exercised them, and compared the results with those in other animals with similar artery narrowing that were not exercised. In the exercised animals, collateral formation was significantly greater.

Then why isn't exercise used in treating angina?

It's beginning to be. Once angina is present, exercise must be taken cautiously. But some new evidence suggests that it can be valuable.

Some physicians work with angina patients in their office. They put the patients through very mild exercise at first and gradually increase the vigor, always stopping just short of what would produce an angina attack. Some even use electrocardiograms during the workouts as a way of anticipating when an angina attack may be coming. Before long, patients learn for themselves just how far they can go in exercising without bringing on angina. And as they keep working out at home, they can gradually go further and further, and they feel better and better.

To participate in one study, twenty-one men with angina gave up work for a month. Each of the men was to measure out a mile course near his home and was to try to walk the mile in twenty minutes four times a day. If chest pain developed, he was to stop immediately and when the pain subsided was to continue more leisurely. When the mile could be completed in twenty minutes without chest pain, he was then to increase his walking pace so he could cover the mile in fifteen minutes. Eventually, he was to get to the point where he could cover the mile in nine minutes by alternately jogging and walking 100 paces. There was very close medical supervision. At the end of the month the patients were enthusiastic about how much better in general they felt. And as the program continued, fifteen of the twenty had complete relief of chest discomfort on exertion.

Is exercise being used after actual heart attacks?

It wasn't so long ago that people who had had heart attacks were consigned to invalidism. Now many physicians encourage selected heart patients to start slowly and move progressively toward vigorous exercise.

One of the pioneering programs in this country has been going on for some years in Cleveland. A prize example there is a man who, one year after his heart attack, was able to run almost five miles in thirty-nine minutes.

Programs for rehabilitating heart patients carried out abroad have produced some striking evidence of the value of exercise. In one program in Israel, patients who have had heart attacks start out with mild exercises for several months. After about nine months, they start to hike, swim, row, run, cycle. Finally they participate in competitive team games. This particular program has been established since 1955—long enough to really see results. Of more than 1,000 heart patients taking part, only 40 have died of heart trouble. Their death rate from heart disease has been less than one-third that of comparable heart patients who did not participate and remained physically inactive.

Apart from circulation, doesn't exercise put a strain on the heart itself?

No. Exercise can make the heart more efficient as well as stronger. What happens when you exercise any muscle? You make it grow and make it stronger and it then does its work more efficiently. The same with the heart. A trained athlete's heart is enlarged because the muscle fibers gradually enlarge. Because they enlarge, the ventricles of the heart enlarge and can hold and pump more blood.

When an athlete is resting, his heart empties only partially with each beat; it doesn't have to pump out all its blood. Moreover, because physical activity has spurred collateral vessel formation, the heart muscle is fed more efficiently. And physical activity also increases blood channels to the exercised muscles so they have a greater ability to extract oxygen from a given amount of blood.

Because of all of this, the heart rate of an athlete at rest may be as little as half that of a more sedentary person. Because the larger heart doesn't have to beat as often when the individual is at rest there are increased rest periods between beats.

During vigorous activity the athlete's heart responds readily. It can contract more completely with each beat to pump out more blood each time than it does when at rest. In an untrained person, increased activity means the heart has to beat more often. But in the trained person the extra blood that can be pumped out with each beat means that the heart rate doesn't have to jump so high. And once the activity is over, the heart rate of a trained person slows down again far more quickly than that of an unfit individual.

Can exercise help the heart in any other ways?

After working with rats, investigators at the University of Pittsburgh School of Medicine first reported to an American Heart Association meeting in 1970 that physical training enabled the hearts of animals to contract with greater force and to deliver more blood per squeeze than hearts of sedentary rats. One reason was the greater ability of coronary blood vessels in the conditioned rats to deliver more oxygen and nutrients to the heart muscle.

At a 1971 meeting the same investigators went further. They had had one group of rats swim 90 minutes a day for four, six, or eight weeks. Another group swam 150 minutes a day for eight weeks. Upon sacrifice, the hearts of the rats in the two groups were compared with those of rats whose only exercise was normal cage activity.

The comparisons showed that physical conditioning alters the chemistry of the heart. In the autopsied hearts of the active rats, the investigators found more of a protein factor called actomyosin ATPase. This substance acts to set off the fuel (ATP) needed for heart muscle contraction. With more of this chemical available, the heart muscle can pump with more force. The amount of ATPase was higher in the active rats, and the greater the duration and intensity of the physical conditioning program, the greater the amount of ATPase.

Is it possible to tell how fit an individual is by what his pulse rate is?

The pulse reflects the beat of the heart. When the heart contracts and forces blood into the aorta, the aorta expands, and a wave of expansion moves along the artery walls branching off the aorta. This happens every time the heart beats.

A simple way to take the pulse is to hold the palm of the left hand up, then place the tip of the right-hand index finger on the outer part of the upturned left wrist, very near the wristband of your watch, if you wear one. You should feel a firm throb of the pulse; if not, move the fingertip until you can feel it.

Often a trained athlete will have a resting pulse rate below 50 per minute. For a man in good condition, it should be less than 70. For a woman, a value below 75 is good. If the rate is faster, it could mean daily physical activities aren't sufficient to keep the heart in good trim. Something else, however, may have to be considered. In some people a high pulse rate stems from excessive use of coffee, tobacco, or alcohol.

Another test is to take the pulse immediately after standing quietly in one place for two or three minutes. If it increases more than 15 beats a minute over the resting pulse rate, or goes above 100, it indicates poor condition.

A third check, if you come through the first two well, is to carry out some mild exercise, such as running in place, for about a minute, then lie down and immediately take the pulse. If the rate is above 100 a minute, your physical condition may be under par.

Can the pulse rate be used as a predictor of trouble?

It can be used that way, according to some studies. They suggest that the resting pulse rate may indicate a greater or lesser likelihood of heart attack and of death from other causes.

In the Framingham study, the death rate from heart attacks was almost four times greater for men and women with pulse rates over 92 than for those with rates less than 67. Other investigations indicate that a rate above 90 per minute adds to the risk of death in people who are obese or have high blood pressure.

One long-term study in Chicago has been covering 1,329 men employed by a large company. They were forty to fifty-nine years old and free of coronary heart disease at the start of the study in 1958. The resting pulse rate was under 70 for 603 men; 70 to 78 for 480; 80 to 89 for 161; and more than 90 for 85 men. The ten-year mortality rate per 1,000 for sudden death has ranged from eight in the men with lowest pulse rate to 41 in those with highest pulse rate; for death from coronary heart disease, from 33 to 82; and for deaths from all causes, from 98 to 211.

Any other benefits to be expected from exercise?

It strengthens muscles, of course, and increases endurance. It may also increase coordination and joint flexibility. In doing that, it may reduce the incidence of minor aches and pains. Many people who've slumped into a state of chronic listlessness and fatigue have, when they could bring themselves to engage in some kind of regular physical activity, found that they felt more alert and energetic. Exercise can be useful in correcting postural defects, and it's likely to produce some improvement in general appearance.

Today exercise is used to treat a considerable variety of ailments. Emphysema is one. At the National Jewish Hospital and Research Center in Denver, exercise constitutes almost the entire treatment program for this serious, increasingly prevalent lung disease that makes thousands invalids yearly. Patients are first taught exercises to help them bring up mucus from their lungs so they cough it out. Then they are taught to breathe a new way, by using large rib muscles to do work the lungs no longer do well. Finally they are taught body-building exercises.

Asthma is also benefited by exercise. At the National Jewish Hospital, younger asthma patients exercise regularly by playing basketball, soccer, softball, and football. In Sweden, juvenile asthmatics who formerly would have been excused from school sports, are playing ice hockey and basketball and following a strenuous physical-training program. Swedish researchers report that such activity is paying high physical and psychologic dividends.

Many physicians now consider exercise valuable in diabetes treatment. It burns up excess sugar in the blood, and helps reduce insulin needs.

Orthopedic problems respond well to exercise. Exercise is used for physical deformities and dysfunctions caused by accidents, birth defects, and strokes. Many physicians urge patients with low-back pain to exercise in order to strengthen weak muscles and relax those that are too tense.

Any claims that exercise can make one young again?

There's beginning to be some scientific evidence it may, at least in some ways.

Men in their seventies, for example, may regain much of the vigor of the forties through carefully planned exercise, according to Dr. Herbert deVries of the University of Southern California. His research at USC's Gerontology Center seeks to learn whether exercise can slow down aging, and what kind of exercise and how much is beneficial. This is one of several projects in American universities and hospitals that seek answers to these basic questions.

Although deVries's work is far from finished, he believes that results so far indicate that exercise has both preventive and therapeutic value and that it may prolong life by slowing the aging process. Taking part in his long-term study are 160 oldsters, ranging in age to eighty-seven, who are given prescribed exercises. In less than a year, they show this kind of average improvement: blood pressure lowered by 6 percent, body fat by 4.8 percent, maximum oxygen consumption (a good objective measure of vigor) up by 9.2 percent; arm strength up by 7.2 percent. DeVries also reports that one of the most significant changes has been a startling drop in nervous tension.

One of DeVries's long-range goals is to build up a "pharmacopoeia of exercise," a reference book physicians could use to get information on the kind and amount of exercise to prescribe for a specific individual based on findings in a physical examination. DeVries believes it will not be long before physicians will prescribe exercise with the same detail and exactness as they now use in prescribing drugs.

When it comes to obesity, is the best diet exercise?

That's carrying it a bit far, but not much. Exercise is important in regulating body weight. Consider how farmers treat hogs: When they want to fatten them, they pen them up.

Of course, obesity is the end product of many influences. Some are constitutional. Certain body types are likely to become obese, others not. Constitutional factors are complex; they may have to do with how brain centers function in regulating appetite and satiety, and how fat tissue is metabolized.

But to no small extent obesity for most people is a problem analogous to hog fattening. We have plenty to eat and an abundance of concentrated calories, from pies to martinis. We are also penned up in a world where physical labor generally has become unnecessary.

Actually, the increase in the problem of obesity has taken place despite a slow reduction in the consumption of food calories per capita. We don't eat as much as our pioneering forefathers did and not as much as people did a century ago. So if we're growing fat, it must be because activity has decreased.

But there's still a lot of misunderstanding about exercise and obesity. Exercise has been ridiculed on the basis that it consumes very little energy. Horrible examples are often cited: to get rid of a pound of fat you have to play handball for eleven hours or split wood for seven hours. Hardly anybody but a lumberjack—and only one in top shape—is likely to split wood for seven hours.

But why assume that exercise has to be done in a single long session? Split wood for just fifteen minutes a day and in a year you will be rid of thirteen pounds of fat. Or play handball for half an hour a day and you will lose sixteen pounds in a year. Or bicycle for half an hour a day and you will lose more than thirty pounds in a year.

Doesn't exercise bring on increased hunger?

Some people say that exercise is self-defeating; that the more you exercise, the more you eat. But it doesn't inevitably work that way. There's a difference between fat people and normal people and the effect of exercise on the appetite of both types.

A person of normal weight in good condition will tend to eat more after increased activity. That, in fact, is why the weight of most normal people tends to remain relatively constant. But the obese person does not react the same way. Only when he exercises to excess will his appetite increase. Because he has plenty of stored fat, moderate exercise does not stimulate his appetite. The difference in response to exercise between fat and normal people is important.

Animal tests have shown that when exercise is moderate, eating does not increase. In one study animals exercised an hour a day ate a smaller amount of food than animals not exercised at all. On the other hand, when the animals were exercised vigorously over longer periods, they ate more but the extra activity kept their weight constant.

Dr. Jean Mayer and other Harvard investigators studied obesity among public school children in two Massachusetts cities. They found that most weight was gained during the winter, the season of least physical activity.

Are fat people generally less active than others?

Some of the most striking studies on activity levels were done with schoolgirls by Mayer and his Harvard group.

They compared food intake and activity schedules of obese and normal girls and found that most of the obese girls actually ate somewhat less, not more, than the normal girls but spent two-thirds less time in physical activity.

Mayer and his group did a thorough analysis of a series of 29,000 short (three-second) motion pictures taken every three minutes of obese and normal girls engaged in a variety of physical activities. They were able to show that the amount of time spent in motion by the obese girls and the caloric cost of these motions were far less than corresponding values for the non-obese. For example, in volleyball, girls of normal weight were motionless on the average half the time but obese girls stood still 85 percent of the time. In tennis, normal girls were motionless 15 percent of the time; obese girls, 60 percent.

Who benefits most from exercise?

Everyone—fat people get thin and thin people keep from getting fat. It takes eating only a few more calories a day than are burned up to have a telling effect in just a few years. One physician, an expert in obesity, likes to put it this way: A woman needs to eat an average of only ninety-six calories a day more than she expends in order to gain fifty pounds from the time of her marriage to the arrival of her third child five years later. Had she added only twenty-five minutes of brisk walking to her daily activities, the weight gain would have been avoided.

The average man will burn up 2,400 to 4,500 calories a day depending on the amount and kind of exercise he gets. Active men—laborers, athletes, soldiers in the field—may consume as many as 6,000 calories a day and not gain weight.

In one experiment a group of university students increased their daily food intake from 3,000 calories to 6,000 calories a day without gaining weight. They did it by stepping up the amount of daily exercise.

Do fat people benefit more from exercise than thin ones?

Only in the sense that it takes more energy to move a heavier body. So for a given amount of time spent in exercise, a fat person may get more benefits in terms of burning up calories. For example, a 100-pound person walking three miles per hour may burn fifty calories in fifteen minutes; someone weighing 200 pounds would use up eighty calories in that time.

Can exercise be dangerous?

You bet it can. Go on a crash program, and it may be the last program of any kind you have a chance to indulge in. Exercise any muscle too vigorously, especially when it has been soft and flabby, and considerable aching is the result. If you overexercise and you are not accustomed to exercise, you may suddenly experience the pain of angina or drop dead. Don't be naïve about exercise.

What's the safe approach to exercise?

First, get a medical checkup. If you pass it, start to exercise slowly—train, don't strain.

A very good way to begin is to walk. Start with a fifteen-minute walk at a relatively leisurely pace. After several days step up the pace, then gradually step up the time. By the time you work up to, say, two daily brisk walking sessions of twenty minutes each, you may find yourself occasionally breaking into a jog briefly just because you feel like it. Have patience. Take it easy. Never push exertion beyond the dictates of common sense.

You can be sure you've overdone it if your heart won't stop pounding for ten minutes after exercising, your breathing is still uncomfortable ten minutes afterward, if you can't sleep well the night after exercising, or if you carry fatigue (not muscle soreness) into the next day.

What are the best exercises?

Don't rely on isometrics, those contraction exercises that work out a muscle by pushing against an immovable object or by pitting one muscle against another for a few seconds. Isometrics can strengthen individual muscles; they may be valuable for that purpose.

But the best overall exercises are those that work out the heart and lungs as well as individual muscles. They involve repetitive movements instead of being static, and they build up endurance and stamina rather than just individual muscle strength. Walking, jogging, running, bicycling, swimming, tennis, volleyball—all fall in this category.

Brisk walking is one of the most valuable but least appreciated forms of exercise. It brings a lot of muscles into play. It stimulates circulation—the massaging action of leg muscles on veins as you walk speeds the return of blood to the heart.

Typical of what walking can do are the results reported from a special study at the Bowman Gray School of Medicine at Winston-Salem, North Carolina. It was carried out with a group of men about fifty years of age who volunteered to participate for forty minutes at a time, four times a week, for twenty weeks. They walked progressively faster until during weeks sixteen to twenty they walked three and one-quarter miles in forty minutes. They showed a 28 percent increase in maximal oxygen intake and a 15 percent increase in pulmonary ventilation (both very good signs of increased vigor). They also had significant reductions in blood pressure, pulse rate, body weight, and body fat.

Golf provides some exercise. Millions of people love the game. If you find in it camaraderie and relaxation, that's all to the good. If you make the course circuit by walking, not riding in a go-cart, you get exercise. Since the walking is not continuous, there is less opportunity to build stamina. So, usually, golf cannot be relied upon as the prime source of exercise. But it can be a pleasant, helpful additional source.

Tennis provides plenty of exercise for legs, heart, and lungs. It can be a delightful sport, provided your physician thinks it's OK for you, and you start slowly.

Swimming, jogging, and bicycling are all excellent because they don't call for any sudden tremendous effort. Like walking, they allow you to start slowly and progress at a healthy pace.

Swimming is fine if you have access to a pool and can swim several times a week as a practical matter.

There is much to be said for jogging. It's an inexpensive sport; there are no club dues and no expensive apparatus to buy. And it can be engaged in day or night.

Bicycling is becoming increasingly popular. Since the mid-fifties, bicycles in the United States have doubled to an estimated 43 million, one for every 2.4 registered cars. Steady pedaling can keep you as physically fit as jogging, and you may find it less monotonous. You can keep in shape with three or four sessions a week, each half an hour to an hour, starting easily. Indoor cycling is useful. So is running in place indoors.

What about other sports?

Fishing is wonderful for relaxation, but it hardly provides a solid dose of strength- and stamina-building activity. Bowling provides only intermittent effort and can't be relied upon as a prime source of exercise. Under usual circumstances, however pleasant, sailing does not provide enough sustained activity to be a prime source. Rowing and canoeing, however, do provide opportunities for exertion, with the amount of exertion controllable, and with a chance to progress at your own rate.

Doesn't exercise take time?

Sure. But not an excessive amount. And it's a remarkably sound investment of time. By giving an hour or two a week to exercise, you may add years to your useful life. If, in a daily workout, you expend some 2,000 extra heartbeats, you're conditioning your heart so that the rest of the day you may save 10,000 to 30,000 beats.

Are exercise gadgets of any value?

To their manufacturers, undoubtedly. Only a few are really useful to the people who use them.

It has been reported that the fitness industry in the United States is a $200-million-a-year business. Never before has the American paunch faced such an awesome array of so-called health hardware, a lot of it expensive, ranging from $195 jogging treadmills to "exercise masters" at $450.

"The beauty of this business," chortles one manufacturer quoted in a business journal account of the industry, "is that nobody really needs this stuff. If he really wants to get into shape, all he needs is a $13.95 sweat suit and some $6.95 sneakers and start running around the block. But people have a great desire for things they don't need. It's marvelous."

On the other hand, some in the industry argue that anyone who invests $400 or $500 in equipment has an "awful lot of incentive to exercise."

If you want to buy equipment like an indoor cycle or any

other apparatus that calls for active work on your part and some sweating, OK. But many people think they're accomplishing something when they use "effortless exercisers," or various kinds of belts and other wearables supposed to take off pounds. The simple fact is you have to work up a sweat not just to reduce but to also make your exercise periods useful for strengthening heart, lungs, and blood vessels, for reducing elevated blood pressure, elevated cholesterol levels, and for evaporating anxieties and frustrations.

Do women need exercise as much as men do?

Perhaps even more! And they may benefit in even more ways than men! Investigators report that physically active women suffer less from angina and heart attacks, and less from a lot of other problems such as chronic fatigue, backaches, and menstrual discomforts.

After doing considerable research in the area, Dr. Evelyn S. Gendel of the Kansas State Department of Health has advised physicians that "the tired, complaining, cross female companion, date, wife, daughter or friend is no joy to anyone." She may have a physical disorder of course. But if she turns out to be physically normal as she so often does, "then we must, as physicians, develop a higher index of suspicion about her physical fitness."

Dr. Gendel has studied many women, of all ages, including young women just out of college. She reports that those who were physically active had the fewest complaints about colds, allergies, digestive disturbances, and fatigue. Those who were least active had the highest incidence of backache troubles.

In one of her studies of 100 postpregnancy women aged eighteen to twenty-three, Dr. Gendel found that thirty-five, more than a third, had low back pain without any kidney, pelvic, or other pathology. "Underdeveloped abdominal musculature was the common finding. The same women also had histories indicating no regular physical exertion or sports activity since childhood."

12

Diet

*Does some food or class of food have special value
for long life?*

No. But the idea that there is—or should be—has been around
since antiquity. Various kinds of roots, herbs, and oddities such
as snail heads have been proposed as having special virtues. Long
ago in various societies there were strong beliefs about avoiding
the meat of older animals and imbibing the blood of young virgins as means of guaranteeing sexual potency and even guaranteeing rejuvenation. More recently we've had special talents
attributed to royal jelly, garlic pills, apple cider vinegar, black-
strap molasses, brewer's yeast, yogurt, and sea salt.

But don't studies link diet and longevity?

The evidence associates not specific foods but reduced intake
with longer life in animals. The classic studies were those of
Dr. Clive McCay in the 1920s. He divided young rats into two
groups, giving one group a good and balanced diet and as much
as they wanted to eat. They lived normal life-spans, the oldest
living 969 days. McCay gave the second group the same kind of
diet, but much less of it—in fact, not enough calories for normal
development. Their growth rate lagged and was kept lagging for
as long as 1,000 days. In effect, the rats were in virtually a
juvenile state all that time. After that, they were given all the

food they could eat and they quickly grew to normal size. And some of these rats lived as long as 1,465 days.

No one knows the reason behind the results of McCay's experiments, but there is a theory. Very recently, Dr. Roy L. Walford of the UCLA School of Medicine found that cutting calories can slow down the aging process and also prevent cancer in mice. Some of his mice on low-calorie diets have lived to double their normal life-span. They also showed significantly fewer cases of cancer than normally fed animals. Walford believes that somehow the body's immunologic defense system is involved.

Among the most profound changes in the body during aging, it appears, are those in the immunologic system. Walford believes that two things happen: the body's infection-fighting capacity is weakened, and simultaneously the immunologic system loses some of its ability to distinguish between the body's own cells and foreign, potentially dangerous materials such as cancer cells. When aging is slowed, its harmful effects are also slowed: the immunologic system remains keen, recognizes cancer cells, wards them off, and continues to fight infections.

But how does a low-calorie diet affect the immunologic system?

No one knows as yet. But Walford is fairly certain about the best time to go on the diet. For mice it is just after weaning. Theoretically, for humans it's at one or two years, not before, since the central nervous system in infants is so immature that calorie deprivation might induce irreversible damage.

Much like McCay's rats, Walford's long-lived cancer-resistant mice received a normal diet after weaning, but at one-third the usual intake; it required a long time for them to mature to full size, but they eventually did. When asked whether his work implies that humans might be wise to eat less, Walford said yes, but the reduced intake should start very young.

Has the human diet been changing?

It keeps changing all the time. Our early ancestors were hunters and food gatherers, who ate fruits, berries, roots, the eggs of both birds and reptiles, and the meat of any small animals they could catch. They were always in search of food, they got plenty of exercise, and they usually could do little more than nibble because they rarely had enough food to stuff themselves. Later, in settled communities, man ate regularly, two or more meals a day, with plenty of starches from cultivated food grains. Early

American settlers ate much protein but also relied heavily on cereals, potatoes, and corn. Until this century, beef wasn't heavily marbled with fat; the livestock were not fattened before slaughter and they were taken long distances to the stockyards.

The American diet today runs about 1,400 pounds of food per person per year on the average, carted home from the markets. That's about 100 pounds less than in the 1940s. But the small can of frozen juice has largely replaced the big bag of fresh oranges and heat-and-eat convenience foods contain less waste. So while take-home poundage is less, it isn't necessarily an indication of ingested poundage.

Meat and potatoes top the list of favored foods in the United States. The average person devours 182 pounds of meat a year, nearly 26 pounds more than a decade ago. And potato intake— 116 pounds a year—is up 9 pounds from a decade ago. On the average, we eat 316 eggs a year, which is 40 fewer than formerly, and consumption of fluid milk and cream, which reached 337 pounds in 1959, is down to 272 pounds for the average person now.

The diet today is supposed to be bad for the heart. There's endless talk about cholesterol. Is diet the whole story?

It's not the whole story, but there is concern about the diet and about changing it in terms of cholesterol and other fatty substances called triglycerides. It's not all a matter of diet by a long shot, but diet is very important.

How does cholesterol fit into the heart picture?

The coronary arteries that nourish the heart muscle are favorite sites for atherosclerosis, a buildup of fatty deposits that may eventually plug an artery and lead to a heart attack.

Cholesterol is believed to be involved. It's a soft, waxy, yellowish substance that is found in every body cell. It plays a role in allowing certain materials to get through cell walls while keeping others out. If, for example, you put your hands in a basin of water, little water soaks into the skin. The reason: Cholesterol in the outer layer of cells makes the skin impermeable to water. Cholesterol also is involved in the production of hormones. The body itself produces this essential material in addition to making use of the supply coming into the body in food. The liver manufactures cholesterol from a chemical, acetyl coenzyme A, derived from fats, carbohydrates, and proteins.

But too much cholesterol circulating in the blood is linked with atherosclerosis. Low blood cholesterol levels are related to low incidence of atherosclerosis and heart attacks, and high levels of cholesterol are found in people with high incidence of disease. Studies in this country show that the higher the cholesterol level, the greater the likelihood of heart attack.

In the Framingham study, for example, coronary heart disease incidence was seven times greater in people with cholesterol above 259 than among those with levels below 200.

But that's guilt by association. What about evidence of cause and effect?

True, the fact that higher cholesterol levels are associated with higher coronary heart disease rates doesn't prove that cholesterol is the cause. But some cause-and-effect evidence comes from animal studies.

More than sixty years ago a Russian scientist showed that if cholesterol was dissolved in vegetable oil and fed to rabbits, artery damage followed. Later, in Chicago, Dr. Louis N. Katz fed cholesterol to chicks and observed similar damage.

Most recently, University of Chicago researchers produced evidence that the typical American diet with its cholesterol load fosters development of atherosclerosis, and that a "prudent" modification of the diet could help avoid artery clogging. They experimented with rhesus monkeys which are much like humans in the way their body metabolism handles various foodstuffs.

Some of the monkeys were given a typical American human diet—milk, eggs, beef, pork, cheese, potatoes, cake, bread, butter, sugar, and so on. Other monkeys on a low-cholesterol "prudent" diet, ate many of the same foods but less or none of those heavily laden with cholesterol and saturated fats, such as eggs, cheese, butter, and fatty beef and pork. The prudent diet also had less sugar and one-third fewer calories than the average American diet.

The monkeys stayed on the diets for two years. Those on the typical American diet had three times as much atherosclerotic disease as those eating the "prudent" diet.

Is there any evidence for humans?

Certain people are born with an inherited tendency to have high blood cholesterol levels. They are particularly prone to atherosclerosis and heart attacks at early ages. It's also been noted that peptic ulcer patients placed on a diet rich in cream and milk and very soothing for ulcers are more subject to heart attacks than other people.

The cholesterol story is not fully known. Cholesterol may or may not be involved in actually triggering atherosclerosis, but most investigators have little doubt that it's involved somehow in the disease process.

Are high cholesterol levels more deadly for women?

Curiously, it appears that women with high cholesterol levels fare even worse than men. Dr. Charles W. Frank of the Albert Einstein College of Medicine recently studied 745 men and 228 women between the ages of twenty-five and sixty-four for three and one-half years after they first developed either anginal chest pain or an actual heart attack. In that time, as compared with the men, the women had a significantly higher probability of getting a first heart attack if they already had angina, or of getting another heart attack if they already had had one. They also had a greater chance of dying from a heart attack.

What is a normal cholesterol level?

That's still undetermined. The problem is that if you take an overall average for Americans, you may come up with a figure such as 250. That means 250 milligrams of cholesterol in 100 milliliters of blood serum. But if that's average, is it normal? Not necessarily normal—not any more than an average weight, a figure that includes all the fatties, is normal or desirable. A value of 150 is not uncommon among many peoples in other parts of the world who have a much lower incidence of heart attacks than Americans.

Most physicians would consider that people with a 200 value are fortunate. But at least one American authority on cholesterol considers that 180 is the upper limit of normal and believes that a true normal would be much lower.

What's a cholesterol test like?

Much like any other blood test. It is usually done before breakfast after an overnight fast. A blood sample is taken from a vein and, in the laboratory, the serum or liquid part is separated out and chemically analyzed.

Since there can be some day-to-day differences in an individual's cholesterol level, the test may be repeated another day, particularly if a first test shows a borderline value.

How can one reduce a high cholesterol level?

Sometimes drugs may be needed to reduce cholesterol level. Usually it can be done with diet alone. But it's not simply a matter of eliminating all cholesterol in the diet, even if that were possible. Cholesterol is present in virtually all foods. It's particularly concentrated in such items as egg yolk, butter, cream, cheeses of various kinds (except dry cottage cheese), sweetbreads, calf brains, and shrimp. In a three-and-a-half-ounce portion of butter, for example, there are 249 milligrams of cholesterol; in an equivalent portion of cream, 140; shrimp, 161; cheeses, 33 to 157. And the cholesterol content in egg yolks is 1370 and in calf brains 1810. If cholesterol is high, one should eat sparingly of such items. But that wouldn't be enough.

The body can make cholesterol out of many foods, for the liver is a highly productive cholesterol factory. Saturated fats in the diet tend to raise the level of cholesterol in the blood. Saturated fats are the fats that harden at room temperature. They occur in beef, lamb, pork and ham; in butter, cream, and whole milk; and in cheeses made from cream and whole milk. They are also found in many solid and hydrogenated shortenings and in coconut oil, cocoa butter, and palm oil (used commercially to make cookies, pie fillings, and nondairy milk and cream substitutes).

What are the so-called polyunsaturated fats?

The term "polyunsaturated" means "highly unsaturated." Saturation is a chemical term relating to the hydrogen content of fats. If a fat is loaded with all the hydrogen it can hold, it's saturated. If it can take on a little more hydrogen, it's slightly unsaturated, and the more it can take on, the more unsaturated it is.

Polyunsaturated fats tend to lower blood cholesterol levels by helping the body to eliminate excess newly formed cholesterol. They are usually liquid oils of vegetable origin such as corn, cottonseed, safflower, sesame seed, soybean, and sunflower seed oils. Olive and peanut oils are also vegetable in origin but are low in polyunsaturated fats; they neither raise nor lower blood cholesterol.

A practical approach for many people with elevated cholesterol levels involves what might be called multiple moderation: much less use of high-cholesterol foods, somewhat lower intake of fats, particularly unsaturated fats, and some use of polyunsaturated fats.

In 1957, the New York City Health Department established an Anticoronary Club to determine whether a change in eating could reduce cholesterol levels and the risk of coronary heart disease. The department's Bureau of Nutrition developed what came to be known as the "prudent diet." It was designed to moderate fat intake and also to equalize saturated and unsaturated fats.

Fish, rich in polyunsaturates, was to be eaten at least five times a week; beef could be eaten only four times; the remaining lunches and dinners were to include veal or poultry. Vegetables and fruits, cereals, and vegetable oils were fine, but only four eggs a week and no butter, ice cream, or hard cheese were allowed. Low-saturated-fat margarines, sherbet, and cottage cheese were recommended, but no rich desserts or pastries.

Some 900 men, forty to fifty-nine years of age, mostly from managerial and professional occupations, joined the club and went on the diet under close supervision. By 1959 they had proved they could learn to live with and even relish the diet. Within the first six months, blood cholesterol levels dropped, and the higher before the diet, the greater the fall—from 300 to 240, for example, or from 260 to 220.

Later, other men joined up. By 1965 there were enough data for comparisons to be made between the heart attack rate of the dieters and the rate for a control group. There had been only one-third as many heart attacks among the dieters as among the controls.

What's the current status of diet treatment?

The American Heart Association is actively sponsoring, and many physicians are recommending, a fat-controlled, low-cholesterol meal plan to reduce the risk of heart attack. You can get a leaflet from your local Heart Association chapter describing the plan in some detail.

Basically, it controls intake of cholesterol-rich foods by limiting use of shellfish and organ meats and restricting intake of egg yolks to three a week. It controls the amount and type of fat by calling for use of fish, chicken, turkey, and veal in most meat meals for the week, and restricting beef, lamb, pork, and ham to five moderate-sized portions per week. It calls for choosing lean cuts of meat, trimming any visible fat, and discarding any fat that cooks out of the meat. It recommends avoiding deep-fat frying and using cooking methods—baking, broiling, boiling, roasting, stewing—that help to remove fat. It restricts the use of fatty luncheon and variety meats such as salami and sausages; calls for use of liquid vegetable oils and margarines rich in polyunsaturated fats in place of butter and other solid or completely hydrogenated cooking fats; and recommends skimmed milk and skimmed-milk cheeses instead of whole milk and whole-milk cheeses.

What are triglycerides?

A triglyceride is a combination of glycerol with three fatty acids. Triglycerides are common in butter, cream, many meats, and most fatty foods. Actually, triglycerides are the main form in which fat is found in the body, both fat stored in the tissues and fat used in producing energy. Like cholesterol, triglycerides are always present in the blood. And, just as with cholesterol, a marked rise in triglyceride blood levels may be associated with coronary heart disease.

Do triglycerides affect cholesterol, or vice versa?

In 1956 Dr. Margaret J. Albrink, now at West Virginia University School of Medicine and then at Yale, first reported a link between triglyceride concentration and coronary heart disease. She noted that as cholesterol went up, so did triglycerides, and that more than 70 percent of men with cholesterol over 260 also had high levels of triglycerides.

Soon other investigators picked up the trail. In 1965 results of one long-term study indicated that both cholesterol and triglycerides are important. For any given cholesterol level, the coronary risk increased with increases in triglycerides, and vice versa. This had also been found in the Framingham study. In addition, the Framingham study found that people with high levels of both cholesterol and triglycerides seemed to be worse off than people who had high levels of only one or the other. This suggested that cholesterol and triglycerides each had an independent effect.

What causes abnormal triglyceride levels?

A major culprit seems to be weight gain. Apparently at about age twenty-five many men go from an active life to a more sedentary one. Marriage may have something to do with that. "The acquisition of a good cook and the security of married life," says Dr. Albrink, "are frequently followed by an abrupt gain in weight by young adult men." She advocates weight reduction as a treatment for elevated triglycerides.

Excess sugar intake may also be involved, either because of the excess itself or because some people are particularly sensitive to it.

Some investigators have a theory that the changing diet in modern times in advanced countries—the change toward more fat and sugar consumption—may account for the increase in coronary heart disease. Some even believe that the increased sugar consumption may be more responsible than the increased fat consumption.

Are we really using so much more sugar?

Sugar was very much of a luxury until the nineteenth century, when it was refined from beets and came into common use. It's been estimated that in England average consumption increased sixfold in the nineteenth century and today runs about 2.3 pounds per person per week.

The average American, it's estimated, may eat at least that much and maybe as much as three pounds a week. That's a startlingly high figure, maybe much too high. But a lot of sugar is consumed these days, in beverages, on cereals, in pies, cakes, jellies, jams, ice cream, and even in some soups, vegetable juices, and salad dressings.

What damage does the excess sugar do?

Dr. John Yudkin of England is one of the leading proponents of the sugar-culprit theory. Based on his studies, he believes that people, on the whole, who eat more than one-quarter pound a day are five times as likely to develop heart attacks as those eating less than one-seventh pound. Not all people, though, he notes, are sensitive to sugar. His findings suggest that about one-third of all people are specially sensitive and develop high triglyceride levels when they eat large amounts of sugar.

In this country, Dr. Peter Kuo of the University of Pennsylvania has found that most people with heart disease and high triglyceride levels are sensitive to excess sugar.

Sugar is carbohydrate; so is starch. The body normally converts some excess carbohydrate calories into fats. It appears that in atherosclerosis-prone people, the conversion is exaggerated. A lot of their excess carbohydrate calories turn to fat.

Most people are more likely to get an excess of carbohydrates from sugar than from starches, some investigators point out. For example, a single chocolate bar is the equivalent of half a dozen slices of bread.

Many people, Dr. Kuo has found, have high blood fat levels that are carbohydrate-sensitive. Their high levels are reduced when they are placed on diets restricting sugar as well as saturated fats.

Is there more than one problem regarding fat in the blood?

Actually, five different types of problems have been classified, which represents a major medical advance. It means that if you have hyperlipidemia (elevated blood fats), the type can be tested for and treated specifically.

What are the types?

The person with type I has only slightly elevated cholesterol but greatly elevated triglyceride levels. Type I is rare. It appears to result from an inherited deficiency of an enzyme. An individual who has it may suffer repeated abdominal pain attacks and skin outbreaks associated with eating fats. On a low-fat diet in which no more than 20 percent of total caloric intake is made up of fats, the triglyceride level comes down and the attacks and outbreaks may disappear.

Type II is more common. Here cholesterol is up but triglycerides are not. One cause is excessive cholesterol intake. Type II also can stem from kidney disorder, liver disease, or thyroid disease, and treatment for the causative disease lowers the cholesterol level. If none of these diseases is present, it's a good bet that the person's mother or father and half his brothers, sisters, and children have the same pattern. Diet treatment—reduction of cholesterol intake with avoidance of eggs, many dairy products, and fatty meats and increased use of unsaturated fats— often helps. When that's not enough, a cholesterol-lowering drug may be used.

In type III, which like type I is not very common, both cholesterol and triglyceride blood levels are up and the risk of early coronary heart disease is great. People with type III are often overweight, and diet treatment calls not only for reducing cholesterol intake but also for weight reduction through reduced caloric intake and a balanced diet. In some cases, a drug called clofibrate may be used.

Type IV is common. Cholesterol may be normal but triglyceride levels are up. A large number of people with coronary heart disease fall into this category. Many are overweight. Diet treatment aims at reducing weight to ideal, reducing carbohydrate intake, and increasing the amount of unsaturated fats used. A diet regimen often is effective in itself. Clofibrate or other drugs may be used if needed.

Type V may run in families, or it may be associated with diabetes, kidney disease, or alcoholism. Sometimes cholesterol level is only a bit high; sometimes it's very high. Always triglyceride levels are way up. People with type V appear to have low tolerance for dietary fat and may need a diet high in protein and low in fats and carbohydrates. Clofibrate or other medication may be used.

Can anybody be tested for type?

The test, made on a blood sample, is more complicated than some others, but it's quickly becoming routine in many hospital and commercial laboratories. If your physician decides you need one, you can get one. If a familial pattern becomes apparent, other members of the family can be tested and treated if necessary.

What kinds of drugs reduce blood fats?

Quite a few different substances have an effect. A vitamin called nicotinic acid in large doses cuts cholesterol levels. Unfortunately, it causes severe blushing and nausea in some people.

Thyroid compounds are sometimes used. People with overactive thyroid glands often have low cholesterol levels and those with underactive thyroids often have high cholesterol levels. Thyroid hormone apparently plays a role in regulating blood cholesterol. The natural thyroid hormone, levothyroxine, is potent; it speeds the heart rate. A less potent synthetic form of the hormone, called dextrothyroxin, produces less stimulation for the heart and, some physicians report, is useful in lowering cholesterol.

Certain resins have been developed to combine with cholesterol from food right in the intestine; then the cholesterol, instead of being absorbed, is expelled in the feces. The resins may have another effect; the bile acids coming into the intestine to aid in digestion contain a compound that enters into the body's manufacture of cholesterol. The resins seem to combine with some of this compound and allow it to be expelled in the feces.

Interestingly enough, there's something in apples that may help. Pectin is a soft, slippery substance contained in apples and also in orange rinds. There are reports that pectin may produce a modest decrease in cholesterol levels. Its action may resemble that of the resins, combining with cholesterol and bile acid materials in the gut and allowing them to be expelled in the feces.

How effective is clofibrate?

Clofibrate is among the most promising of any drugs tried thus far. Clofibrate is taken by mouth in capsule form and it reduces both cholesterol and triglyceride blood levels in as many as 80 percent of patients.

How it works is not known definitely. It appears to be safe, but there can be undesirable reactions. About 5 percent of patients taking it experience nausea. Other effects reported less often include vomiting, diarrhea, dyspepsia, and flatulence. These effects often disappear with continued treatment.

Are heart attacks actually reduced?

According to the results of a recent study of more than 3,000 men, clofibrate reduced the heart attack rate by more than two-thirds. In more than 1,000 men whose average age was 47.5 years, the heart attack rate was 1.89 per 1,000 per year for men treated with the drug; it was 6.6 per 1,000 per year for untreated men. The difference was even more striking when more than 2,000 men were tested whose average age was ten years younger. Treated, their heart attack rate was .64 per 1,000 per year; untreated, it was 5 per 1,000 per year.

A very curious finding emerged from the study. The drug did protect men from heart attack when it lowered blood fat levels; but it also protected some men whose fat levels did not come down with treatment. This finding suggests that clofibrate may have another beneficial effect that as yet is unknown.

What generally constitutes a good diet?

You hear a lot about balanced and varied diets, and both balance and variety are important. Take the matter of balance first. Because muscles, heart, liver, kidneys, and many other organs are chiefly protein in composition, proteins from meat, fish, skimmed milk, and other sources are needed for organ development and growth in childhood and youth and later for repair and replacement.

Because bones are made up chiefly of minerals such as calcium and phosphorus, these minerals are needed for growth and then maintenance. One good source is skimmed milk; others are cereals, meat, fish, turnip tops, dandelion greens, and other vegetables.

Carbohydrates are needed for energy. Fats and proteins also supply energy, but less quickly; they can be stored for use as reserves. Sugar can be said to be the fuel of life. It doesn't have to be ingested as table sugar; for in the body starches are quickly converted to sugar, which is burned to supply energy.

Vitamins help convert foods into skin, bones, muscles, nerves, and other body tissues. Only tiny amounts are needed, but they're essential.

All told, nearly fifty different nutrients—including the various amino acid constituents of protein, carbohydrates, vitamins, minerals, fats—are known to be needed for health. A balanced diet can supply them all. For balance, it's generally agreed that foods should be selected each day from each of four basic groups: milk and milk products; cereals and breads; fruits and vegetables; and meat and protein-rich foods (including nuts and dried beans and peas).

However, if you always choose the same foods, you may not be eating an optimum diet.

The fact is that if we now know almost fifty essential nutrients, there could be many more that are still unknown. For example, knowledge about trace elements (discussed in an earlier chapter) is new and still fragmentary. We know that zinc supplements, for example, speed healing of surgical wounds and chronic skin ulcers, but why was there any deficiency of zinc?

Trace elements occur in water and soils, get into foods, may occur in relatively large amounts in some foods, in small amounts or not at all in others. Existing knowledge is scanty. Some trace elements in proper amounts may be beneficial, even essential; some, in abnormal amounts, may be dangerous. Currently science is striving to learn how health is influenced by trace elements, including chromium, cadmium, manganese, cobalt, copper, selenium, molybdenum, vanadium, and nickel. Preliminary evidence suggests that chromium deficiency may play a role in diabetes, while an excess of cadmium may have an unhealthy effect on blood pressure.

Until a lot more is known, it is only sensible to eat a varied as well as balanced diet, picking from a wide variety of foods rather than concentrating on just a few. That way there is a reasonably good chance that you will get most or all of the nutrients, known and unknown, that you need and not too much of any that may be harmful in excess.

What's the most common nutritional deficiency?

Iron, by far, particularly among women. Iron is essential because it is a constitutent of hemoglobin, the pigment that is carried in the red blood cells and transports oxygen. Without enough iron, anemia develops. An amount of iron no bigger than one-fifth of an ounce, the usual body content, stands between each of us and suffocation.

About 1 milligram of iron is lost daily in urine, sweat, and cast-off cells. The average modern diet provides 10 to 15 milligrams daily but only 1 to 1.5 milligrams are absorbed into the body tissues. So the margin of safety is quite narrow.

There's little likelihood of iron deficiency occurring in men unless they bleed internally from an ulcer or other source. Men tend to have a higher caloric intake and so tend to get more iron. But women lose iron in menstrual blood throughout the childbearing years and also eat less and therefore tend to take in less iron than men do. It's estimated that as many as 20 percent of all women of childbearing age are deficient in iron and that adolescent girls, with their often flighty eating habits, get on the average 30 percent less iron than they need.

What foods are rich in iron?

Meats, dry beans, nuts, and most green vegetables are good sources of iron. Many breakfast foods are highly fortified with iron. For women with very high iron requirements because of pregnancy or because of abnormal menstrual losses physicians may prescribe supplemental iron preparations.

What's the reason for abnormal food cravings?

Very often, iron deficiency may cause such cravings. They are particularly common in women, but they occur in men, too. One craving that occurs in both men and women is for ice—two, three, or more trays of cubes daily. Provide the iron they need, and these people stop chewing on ice.

Iron has also been used to cure women of the habit of eating clay and dirt. Many women, especially in the southern states, crave clay during pregnancy and some eat it at other times. In the South, white clay is considered a delicacy, but women eat both white and red varieties. The clay holes are often located in secluded rural spots near railroad beds and rivers or creeks. Their exact whereabouts are often closely guarded secrets. The women often go to unusual lengths to camouflage the holes, which sometimes are so deep the women have to be lowered by their heels to claw for a fresh supply. Many women tell their doctors that they eat their fill of clay during their visit to a hole, but some have been seen popping marble-size balls of clay into their mouths while waiting for appointments with physicians.

Investigators have found that the iron in clay is unusable by the human body. In addition, clay may act as a filter in the gut and absorb the iron from food, so that the more clay eaten, the less iron absorbed in the blood.

But the practice goes on. Boxes of clay are even shipped to relatives in large northern cities, according to Duke University investigators. And many women who live in urban centers where clay is not available have turned to laundry starch.

Are natural foods the most healthful?

There's no simple answer to that question. Organic and unprocessed natural foods are now being widely offered in health-food stores and supermarkets. But authorities now and again find so-called natural foods that aren't natural at all, just labeled as such. If natural foods become more popular, mislabeling may become so, too; it would be difficult if not impossible to supply a very great demand for natural products.

True natural foods—those grown without chemicals and offered with a minimum of processing—are healthful and nutritious. Since they often cost more, the question is whether they are necessary.

They're particularly good, it's claimed, because they are grown in rich rather than impoverished soil and aren't spoiled by processing.

But there are arguments that agriculture in this country generally is oriented toward keeping soil rich through crop rotation and fertilization. There are also arguments from nutrition experts that, for all practical purposes, fresh produce is not superior nutritionally to canned and frozen foods.

Do food additives constitute a danger?

There may be some element of risk, but there is no evidence that it's a great risk.

A lot of food additives are used, including vitamins and minerals, flavoring agents, preservatives to prevent spoilage by microorganisms or undesirable chemical changes, emulsifiers to ensure fineness of grain in bakery goods, and stabilizers and thickeners for texture and body.

Current laws call for many test procedures to establish safety before new additives can be used. Still, a lot remains to be learned about additives and as it's learned more tests may become possible.

Unless ways are found to grow enough natural foods and get them to the table quickly and without processing to feed growing millions, we're going to have to live with additives and with pesticides as well, and find out how to pick the best of them and use them to ensure the most safety.

Can taste be depended upon as a guide to healthy eating?

It's often said that if people—even children—just eat what they feel like eating, they'll eat well and get everything they need: Their taste will guide them. This might be true if eating were done in a vacuum and if taste were not so easily influenced by all kinds of things—not just foods themselves but talk about food, family eating patterns, peer eating patterns, social customs, and a lot more.

Take a look, for example, at the typical teen-age taste in eating. The average teen-ager eats often enough—about five meals a day. The menu includes hamburgers, french fries and catsup, snacks such as potato chips and carbonated beverages, and precious little else, say authorities. According to Dr. Roy Morse, of the Rutgers University Food Science Department, teen-agers have an almost endless number of ways to worry their parents—their hair length, their school grades, their politics, their language, their musical taste, *and* their malnutrition.

But teen-agers aren't alone in lacking nutritional common sense. Many men, full grown and intelligent, are meat-and-potatoes men; no vegetables, or vegetables only occasionally on a sufferance basis. Some women only pick at meat and therefore lack proteins.

Taste can develop if given a chance; it can also be inhibited all too readily. A lot of people would enjoy more foods if they allowed themselves to try them.

And something new has turned up recently. For years, doctors have been puzzled by some patients who complain that just about everything tastes bad, or doesn't taste like anything. The phenomenon has been noted in hospitalized patients who complained about food. For a long time, it was thought to be psychological, but now it has been found to be physical. The problem stems from a disorder called idiopathic hypogeusia, which attacks taste and smell. Some victims have decreased ability to taste and smell; some experience obnoxious taste and odor in their food and drink. Already some 3,000 such people have been discovered, and it's expected that there are many more. Physicians find that feeding such people zinc supplements may reverse the taste abnormalities; they therefore speculate that the taste abnormalities stem from mineral deficiency.

13

Smoking, Drinking, Other Matters of Life-Style

Just how much of a gamble does one take by smoking?

A man age twenty-five who doesn't smoke can expect to live 6.5 years more than a man who smokes a pack of cigarettes a day. According to U.S. statistics, an average heavy smoker (two or more packs), who smokes about 750,000 cigarettes during his lifetime, can expect to lose 8.3 years of life (4.4 million minutes), as compared with a nonsmoker. This amounts to almost 6 minutes per cigarette, *a minute of life for a minute of smoking.*

According to recent British studies, heavy cigarette smokers have a 2-in-5 chance of dying before age sixty-five while a non-smoker has a 1-in-5 chance. The heavy smoker cuts in half his chances of surviving beyond sixty-five.

What about pipes and cigars?

Smoking pipes and cigars is more harmful than not smoking at all, but far less harmful than heavy cigarette smoking.

Cigarette tobacco is flue-cured, retains sugars, and burns at higher temperature than pipe and cigar tobacco. The smoke of a cigarette is acid, and nicotine in acid solution is not absorbed in the mouth but in the passages of the lungs, which of course is why cigarettes are inhaled for satisfaction.

Cigar and pipe tobaccos are air-cured, their sugars disappear over long periods of curing, they burn at lower temperatures, their smoke is more alkaline, and nicotine is more readily absorbed in the mouth from alkaline smoke. Therefore there is less need to inhale cigars and pipes for satisfaction.

Just why cigarette smoking is so much more dangerous isn't yet clearly established. It's not simply a matter of nicotine. Research suggests that on the average a cigarette smoker absorbs about 1 milligram of nicotine from each cigarette; a pipe smoker absorbs about 1.65 milligrams from each pipeful, if he does not inhale; and a cigar smoker may without inhaling, absorb as much nicotine from one cigar as a cigarette smoker does from inhaling five cigarettes. It's possible that the increased harmfulness of cigarettes is related to the higher burning temperature of the tobacco or to the composition of the cigarette paper.

What solid evidence is there that cigarette smoking causes lung cancer?

The first suggestion came almost fifty years ago when a physician in England reported that virtually all lung-cancer patients he saw were chronic cigarette smokers. Subsequently, other physicians made similar observations.

This evidence spurred some large-scale studies, one of which involved 40,000 British physicians who were classified by their smoking habits and followed for the next fifty-four months. Light cigarette smokers were found to be seven times as likely to die of lung cancer as nonsmokers; moderate smokers, twelve times as likely; heavy smokers twenty-four times as likely.

A still larger study in the United States covered 187,783 men who appeared healthy at the beginning. Over the next forty-four months, 11,870 died of various causes. Statisticians established that the lung cancer death rate per 100,000 men per year for nonsmokers was 12.8; for smokers of a pack a day, it was 107.8; for smokers of one to two packs, 229.2; for those smoking more than two packs, 264.2.

Until quite recently, statistical studies provided the only real evidence of the relationship between smoking and lung cancer. The trouble was that animals, useful for a lot of other studies, just didn't take readily to smoking. Finally, experimenters were successful in training beagles to smoke. More than ninety dogs were used in a study in which some did not smoke and others were divided into groups placed on schedules of light and heavy smoking. After about two years, half the heavy smokers had died. The remaining dogs were sacrificed and their lungs examined. Tumors were found in 25 percent of the nonsmoking beagles, 58 percent of the light smokers, and 79 percent of the heavy smokers.

What other effects do cigarettes have on the lungs?

Smoking is an underlying cause of chronic obstructive bronchopulmonary disease (COPD), which includes chronic bronchitis and pulmonary emphysema. COPD is a rapidly increasing cause of death. In 1949 the death rate from COPD was 2.1 per 100,000 people; by 1960, 6.0; by 1967, 12.9. The 600 percent increase in eighteen years is startling.

Most patients with COPD are cigarette smokers. Research statistics show that risk of COPD increases with the number of cigarettes smoked, and for smokers of two packs a day the risk is eighteen times as great as for nonsmokers. The value of giving up smoking has been established. Studies in dogs trained to smoke show that smoking produces emphysema and other abnormal changes in the lungs proportional to the dosage of inhaled smoke.

In areas of high pollution, COPD is more prevalent than elsewhere. But in the absence of smoking the correlation between COPD and air pollution is slight, suggesting that the two factors combined—smoking and pollution—may interact to produce higher rates of disease.

Is smoking cigarettes bad for the heart and blood vessels, too?

A disease called Buerger's disease affects small arteries and veins in the extremities, reducing blood flow. If uncontrolled, it produces gangrene; amputation may be required. Even at the turn of the century it was known that patients with this disease benefitted when they stopped smoking. This was one of the first indications of an effect of smoking on arteries.

About the time of World War II, when electrocardiograms were made of 2,400 seemingly healthy men, 50 percent more abnormal tracings showed up in smokers than in nonsmokers, suggesting some association between cigarettes and heart damage.

Then came the big U.S. study on lung cancer and smoking covering the 187,783 men. It also demonstrated a relationship between smoking and heart disease. The death rate from coronary heart disease was more than twice as high for smokers of a pack or more daily as for nonsmokers; and the greater the number of cigarettes smoked and the greater the number of years of smoking, the higher the death rate—for example, it was one-third higher for those who began to smoke before age fifteen than for those who began after age twenty-five.

There have been many studies since. In the Framingham study, the heart attack risk was nearly double in heavy cigarette smokers; there was a threefold excess of sudden deaths among smokers compared with nonsmokers, and the sudden-death risk in heavy smokers was as much as five times greater.

One study of men who already had coronary heart disease showed that those who continued to smoke a pack or more of cigarettes daily died sixteen years sooner, on the average, than the nonsmokers. At the time of death, the average age of heavy smokers was only 47.4 years, compared with 63.2 years for non-smokers.

What exactly does smoking do to the heart?

The complete answer is not known, but it is known that smoke contains many harmful substances. Nicotine, for example, constricts blood vessels, and that can be harmful.

One ingredient of smoke, carbon monoxide, is getting a lot of attention. When carbon monoxide in cigarette smoke is inhaled and enters the bloodstream, it combines with hemoglobin. Hemoglobin is the pigment in red blood cells that serves to carry oxygen from the lungs to all tissues of the body. When carbon monoxide combines with some of the hemoglobin, there is that much less hemoglobin available to carry oxygen. In a person who already has a heart deprived of plentiful oxygen because of narrowed coronary arteries which limit blood flow, a further reduction in oxygen because of carbon monoxide interference could be fatal.

Moreover, recent research indicates that carbon monoxide may actually foster the development of artery hardening. In rabbits, carbon monoxide greatly increases the deposition of cholesterol in arteries.

Does smoking get all the blame for heart trouble?

Absolutely not; it's one of many factors.

The Finns and the Japanese smoke, on the average, just about the same number of cigarettes. But the coronary death rate of the Finns is nine times greater than that of the Japanese. Finns tend to eat a lot of fat; the Japanese eat less. It may be that excessive cigarette smoking is particularly dangerous for people on high fat and cholesterol diets.

Smoking also seems to be particularly dangerous for physically inactive people. For example, a study covering 110,000 people made by the Health Insurance Plan of Greater New York found that while men who smoke are, on the whole, twice as likely to experience heart attacks as nonsmokers, smokers who are physically inactive are three times as likely to experience the attacks as smokers who have been physically active.

Can smoking produce ulcers?

An association was noted forty years ago, but the mechanism has been discovered only through very recent research. It has long been known that smoking reduces the efficacy of antacid treatment once an ulcer is present and slows healing. Now, in studies with dogs, University of Oklahoma researchers have found that nicotine in the blood may remove protection from the duodenum (the first part of the small intestine) by inhibiting acid-buffering secretions from the pancreas and the gallbladder while the stomach's output of hydrochloric acid continues at the usual rate.

Investigators have also shown that duodenal ulcers can be induced when animals are given hydrochloric acid. But when the acid is given with nicotine, the ulcer incidence is pushed from 30 percent to 90 percent.

Is anything else blamed on smoking?

Women who smoke cigarettes spend 17 percent more days ill in bed than women who have never smoked, according to one study. Other studies show that infants born to mothers who smoke weigh 6.1 ounces less than those of mothers who don't smoke. Women who smoke during pregnancy apparently have a significantly greater number of miscarriages, stillbirths, and infant deaths shortly after birth.

The National Clearinghouse for Smoking and Health estimates that each year in the United States there are 11 million more chronic cases of illness than there would be if all people had the same rate of sickness as those who have never smoked. It figures that there are 280,000 more people with heart conditions than there would be if no one smoked, 1 million more cases of bronchitis or emphysema, 1.8 million more cases of sinusitis, and 1 million more cases of peptic ulcer.

What happens physically during smoking?

There is some reduction of appetite along with dulling of smell and taste. Nicotine first causes the adrenal glands to release a hormone that stimulates the nervous system and also releases some sugar from the liver. Therefore there is an immediate "kick," which is followed soon by an opposite effect as the nervous system becomes depressed. The heart rate increases somewhat, as does blood pressure. Small arteries are constricted, reducing blood flow; drops of about five degrees in the temperatures of the fingers and toes have been measured after the smoking of one cigarette.

Smoking inflames mucous membranes of the nose and throat; any physician can identify a smoker by the presence of this inflammation. The membranes normally produce a sticky material (mucus) designed to trap foreign particles in inhaled air. Normally, too, tiny hairlike projections called cilia which line the breathing passages move in a whiplike manner to push the trapped substances upward so they can be swallowed or expectorated, thus keeping the lungs clean. Cigarette smoking slows cilia action and, if continued long enough, destroys the cilia. Some studies have shown that smokers have nine times as great an incidence of respiratory infections as do nonsmokers.

Cigarette smoking also has been found to stimulate release of fatty acids into the bloodstream. This effect may be involved in producing the higher concentrations of blood cholesterol found in smokers. Studies also show that cigarette smoking accelerates blood clotting, produces abnormal changes in the walls of the air sacs in the lungs, and by so doing may add to the work burden of the heart.

How big is the payoff from giving up cigarettes?

The outlook in terms of heart disease is improved, even for those who already have coronary disease as manifested by angina or a previous heart attack. The risk for lung cancer begins to go down about a year after cigarette smoking is given up; by the tenth year it is slightly higher than for those who never smoked. Symptoms of chronic bronchitis and emphysema improve within a few weeks after smoking is abandoned. Of course, lung tissue damaged by emphysema can't be replaced, but progress of the disease is retarded and may even be stopped.

Other dividends include a better sense of taste and smell, less shortness of breath, relief of nasal stuffiness, and escape from the anxiety about smoking that many people feel. There's also an economic reward—a one-pack-a-day smoker spends upward of $150 a year on the habit.

Cigarette smoking is a tough habit to kick, but maybe it's a bit easier than it used to be. It's estimated that about one-fourth of all men and one-fifth of all women who ever smoked have now stopped. Of all physicians who ever smoked, more than half have quit.

What's the best way to quit smoking—
taper off or stop suddenly?

Of those who have successfully stopped, half stopped suddenly and half stopped gradually, according to Dr. Donald T. Frederickson of New York, an expert in the problem of smokers who wish to quit. Both methods work, and the best way for any person is the one that works for him. Frederickson suggests trying gradual tapering off as a starter; small successes give confidence. But some people find it difficult to taper off. If you're one of them, he suggests that you set a stop date; remove all visible signs of the cigarette habit (cigarette packages, ashtrays, lighters, matches, holders) from home and office; store up temporary substitutes such as low-calorie candies, gums, strips of celery, carrots, etc.; and prepare a three-day schedule of constant activity so you have no time to sit around thinking about not smoking. The critical period is the first forty-eight hours; once beyond this, Frederickson finds, you will be well on your way toward becoming a permanent nonsmoker.

Do group sessions help?

Group sessions are helpful in many cases. In many communities group sessions are conducted by various organizations. Encouragement and support from other people in the same predicament bolsters the courage of the new nonsmoker and reinforces his resolve.

Dr. Frederickson, who organized many groups in New York for the New York City Department of Health, thinks groups are valuable for some people who otherwise could not quit. But he also thinks most individuals can stop on their own once they make the decision and are convinced they really must quit.

Are there any particularly helpful tricks?

Physical exercise often helps greatly. It's a mainstay of the stop-smoking clinics of the Seventh-day Adventist church. Smokers are told to take a brisk walk instead of smoking, to get some vigorous exercise daily.

For one thing, exercise helps to dissipate the tension of stopping. Also, it replaces some of the effects of nicotine. Nicotine speeds the heart and contracts blood vessels; the stimulation is much like that from a spurt of adrenaline when you're in a state of fear or anger. It's not good for you, but many people get so used to it they feel unnatural without the nicotine stimulation. Exercise produces some of the same effects in more healthy fashion and can help dull the desire for nicotine.

Some clinics advocate breathing exercises. They suggest that when you feel the need to smoke, you breathe in slowly, filling the lungs as much as possible, then very slowly exhale, and give an extra push to expel the last of the air. For one thing, such breathing relaxes tension a bit. Actually, some researchers believe that when an individual becomes tense, he tends to breathe shallowly, gets too little oxygen, and then experiences a reflex that makes him want to inhale deeply; often this reflex is misinterpreted by smokers as a desire to smoke, when what they really want is more air. So breathing exercises may help by providing added oxygen.

The real experts at stopping smoking are those who have succeeded. The American Cancer Society has collected from former heavy smokers some suggestions you may find helpful:

• "Develop a set of rules as to where you can and cannot smoke. For instance, I made a rule that when I came home at night I could not smoke in my apartment. If I wanted to smoke, my rule said that I had to go to the basement furnace room. This furnace room is extremely hot. For the first couple of days I was dragging myself up and down the stairs several times a night. However, under no circumstances would I break the rule. Finally I gave up in disgust and stayed in my apartment one whole evening without smoking. It worked! I then developed a rule to make it awkward to smoke in another area of my daily routine. It worked again. Eventually I crowded the cigarette out of my life altogether."

• "I bought ten different kinds of cigarettes and placed one of each in my cigarette case. This meant every time I went to light up I had to smoke a different brand. This made smoking very unpleasant."

• "When I went about my business without a cigarette on my person I would be tempted to buy a pack. However, if I carried one cigarette with me it provided a sense of security. I never 'panicked' and was able to resist the temptation to smoke."

• "I avoided making mental promises to myself to have the next cigarette at a particular time. Instead I left things open for a new decision whether or not to smoke. For example, if I were to say: 'I won't have a cigarette now but I will have one when I reach the office,' invariably I would smoke a cigarette as soon as I arrived at the office. On the other hand, if I said to myself: 'I won't have a cigarette now, postponing what I will do when I reach the office until I arrive,' I found it much easier to control the urge to take the next cigarette. Using this approach I was often able to stall off the next cigarette for considerable periods of time."

• "My experience in stopping ten years ago was associated with a 'craving' feeling located in my chest. I have, therefore, recommended on several occasions that people make a very 'hot' (in the sense of 'peppery') soup or bouillon which they can carry around in a small Thermos bottle. When they have an insatiable desire to smoke, they find that the curious burning sensation of having something 'going down' in the upper chest is satisfied by drinking this soup. It also gives them something to do with their hands and their mouth. Recipe: 1 quart tomato juice, ¾ cup lemon juice. Season to taste with several dashes of Tabasco sauce, Worcestershire sauce, salt and pepper. The pepperier the better! Shake well, serve hot or cold."

• "Tell all of your friends that you are going to stop smoking. This kind of public commitment will really help bolster your determination at those critical moments when you may be tempted to weaken."

• "I set the following schedule for smoking. Every day I would postpone the first cigarette by one half hour. In a short time I found I was able to make it to lunch without smoking. For me this was an absolute miracle for I normally smoked at least a pack and a half during the morning hours. I stuck to my schedule and to my surprise I soon found that I was not smoking at all."

• "My approach was to concern myself only with today. Tomorrow would take care of itself. My long-range objective was to get through each day without smoking. My short-range objective was to overcome every urge to smoke during the day. I believe it was keeping my goal limited and realistic that was the greatest help to me. Besides I think I would have panicked if someone said: 'You will never be able to smoke again!' Now this idea doesn't bother me at all. You see, I am no longer a smoker."

What causes the weight gain when smoking is stopped?

The weight gain does not necessarily stem from increased eating, a recent study shows. At Temple University, investigators enlisted the help of seven scientists, all long-time smokers. For science's sake, they agreed to quit smoking, cold turkey, for one month. The morning before they quit, they underwent tests for basic metabolic rates—the rates at which their bodies transformed foods; after the month, they were retested.

The retesting showed that each former smoker's body was chugging along at a slower rate than previously; basic metabolism had slowed, heart rates were down, on the average, by 3 beats a minute, or more than 4,000 beats a day. The former smokers gained an average of six and one-half pounds each. As trained scientists, they carefully noted their eating habits. Only one said he ate more; he also gained the most weight. One did not gain any weight, attributed by him to the fact that he had done a great deal of skiing during the experiment.

The study indicates that there are two kinds of metabolic rates —one for smokers, one for nonsmokers. A smoker who quits will eventually level off to a new metabolic rate; during the transition period he may gain weight even though he eats no more. If he does, experts say, he can tackle the weight problem later; it's not difficult to lick in such cases. If he exercises during the transition period, he may avoid gain.

Suppose one can't quit entirely?

On a statistical basis, there is a safe number of cigarettes— fewer than five a day. But few if any confirmed smokers can drop to that level for any length of time. In Dr. Frederickson's experience, nine out of ten revert to old smoking rates within weeks.

Some people have switched to cigars or pipes. Anything that reduces the amount of inhaled smoke is to the good. There is some risk of mouth cancer from smoking cigars or pipes but, so long as the smoke is not inhaled, overall mortality of cigar and pipe smokers is only a little higher than that of nonsmokers.

Is alcohol a life shortener?

Probably not in moderation. That's the consensus of medical opinion. But excessive consumption is dangerous. There is increasing evidence that in excess, alcohol is much more of a killer than long supposed even by medical men.

In a recent San Francisco investigation, when many deaths attributed to heart and related diseases were put under intensive scrutiny, it turned out that a goodly number had resulted from other causes. Alcoholism was found to be the underlying cause of death in 129 percent more cases than reported. Cirrhosis of the liver was the real cause in 11.1 percent more deaths than had been reported. Physicians, the investigators noted, are naturally reluctant to tag people as being alcoholics; consciously or subconsciously they may try to draw the shades around the deceased and their close relatives. That's part of the story.

Is alcohol connected with many diseases?

New research is identifying more and more alcohol-related diseases. That alcohol can produce cirrhosis—a scarring and degeneration of the liver that may cause it to fail and lead to death—is an old story. But alcohol also affects muscles, including the heart muscle. Although a relationship between chronic alcoholism and heart disease has long been suspected, until recently the heart damage was believed to develop because of liver disease. Recently, however, investigators have found that heart disease can occur in alcoholics who do not have liver disease. It's alcohol in excess, not the liver disease, that produces the heart problem. At Tulane University Dr. George E. Burch has found heart damage uniformly in mice fed large amounts of alcohol. Alcoholic heart disease, it now appears, may be a common problem.

Among other recent findings: A study of 841 tuberculosis patients in a Veterans Administration hospital found that nearly half were alcoholics. Of a group of patients with cancer of the pancreas, 75 percent were alcoholics.

In a large industrial firm a study of 922 employees who were known or suspected problem drinkers found that, compared with nonalcoholics, they had higher incidences of high blood pressure, stomach ulcer, duodenal ulcer, asthma, diabetes, gout, neuritis, cerebrovascular disease, heart disease, and cirrhosis. On the other hand, heavy use of alcohol did seem to protect them against kidney stones.

Is there such a thing as intelligent drinking?

Many physicians believe so. If there is no physical disorder that may be affected adversely by alcohol, many physicians consider a drink or two before dinner, and perhaps a bit more on special occasions, to be no great hazard and perhaps even beneficial.

It's a matter of timing and moderation. The time to drink is not at lunch but at the end of the workday. The cocktail hour, if it involves an unhurried drink or two, can be pleasant and relaxing, drawing a curtain on any tensions of the day and paving the way to relaxed dining and a relaxed evening. This can be all to the good.

What actually happens in the body with excessive drinking?

Alcohol has a diuretic effect, because it inhibits the pituitary hormone that controls fluid excretion. It also dilates blood vessels, and causes a loss of body heat. It irritates mucous membranes, which is one reason for the nausea and vomiting of the hangover. No one has improved on Shakespeare's observation on the sexual effects of alcohol: "... it both provokes and unprovokes. It provokes the desire but unprovokes the performance."

Alcohol is a food containing seven calories per gram, compared with four calories for carbohydrates and protein and nine for fat. It provides only empty calories, those without essential vitamins or proteins. Many heavy drinkers are poorly nourished because excessive alcohol intake can dull the appetite and because it can irritate the stomach lining enough to make the thought of eating become repulsive.

Every part of the nervous system is susceptible to effects of excessive alcohol intake over prolonged periods. The most obvious effect is peripheral neuropathy, with its numbness, pins-and-needles sensations, and weakness in affected limbs; it can be reversed through therapy with vitamin B_1 (thiamine), but this takes up to six months.

Alcohol in excess depresses the bone marrow where red blood cells are formed, which leads to anemia. It can produce acute muscle pain, tenderness, and fluid retention (alcoholic myopathy), especially in the muscles of the legs and the chest cage. In some cases alcoholic hypoglycemia (low blood sugar) occurs; if not properly treated it may produce coma and irreversible neurologic complications.

How big a problem is alcoholism?

No one knows, although alcoholism is ranked, more or less officially, as the fourth most important health problem in the United States, outranked only by heart disease, mental illness, and cancer.

It has often been said that one of every thirteen adult men is an alcoholic; nobody can make a good estimate of how many women are alcoholics, for they come less frequently to public and medical attention.

According to one very recent study of American drinking practices by George Washington University investigators, 68 percent of American adults drink and 12 percent drink heavily. A survey of men aged twenty-one to fifty-nine by University of California researchers indicated that one of every two American men had had some drinking problem within the last three years, and that the problem was considered fairly severe in one out of every three cases.

Why do some people drink to excess?

Alcohol is readily available. It creates a sense of contentment and release from awareness of responsibilities. A few drinks encourage sociability. Most people regard this as a pleasant but temporary experience. When anyone tries to maintain this pleasant state of unreality by continuous drinking, the danger of alcoholism is great.

People vary in their reaction to alcohol, even in their ability to tolerate it at all when they first try a drink. Some stop right there. Others have milder, more pleasant effects. Some can drink, almost from the beginning, relatively large amounts without seeming to be affected; curiously, they're more likely than others to become alcoholic.

From animal studies it appears that anyone can develop tolerance for alcohol. It can be induced in rats in three weeks. It takes longer in humans. After several years the heavy social drinker often notices that, although he drinks more and more, the effects are less than they used to be. He can walk a straight line, talk clearly, carry on business and other activities with blood alcohol levels that would leave a novice unable to stagger. This is what is called pharmacological tolerance. How it develops is still not clear. As tolerance develops, however, there are behavioral changes that may start with irritability and irresponsibility and progress to blackouts, periods when the alcoholics may seem to be functioning normally but for which he has no recall.

Recently, Dr. Jack Mendelson of Harvard University found that alcoholic subjects actually become not less but more anxious, distraught, and depressed as drinking continues. Why then does the alcoholic go on drinking? An amnesia process may be the reason. Objective tests show that short-term memory begins to fail as blood alcohol level rises. And many alcoholics report drinking episodes as they thought they would be rather than as they actually were.

How can one tell if alcoholism is approaching?

Some years ago, Dr. Harry J. Johnson of the Life Extension Institute suggested a few guidelines that seem as good now as then.

> If two or three years ago, you set aside a half hour for a drink but now the time has stretched to two hours and four drinks. . . .

> If two or three years ago, you looked forward with pleasure to dinner but now there is little interest in food. . . .

> If two or three years ago, you took cocktails at lunch only for business entertaining but now one or two are routine. . . .

> If two or three years ago, weekend consumption was little more than that on weekdays but now drinking starts early in the day, perhaps even in the morning, and continues more or less all day. . . .

If this is your experience, alcoholism is imminent if not already present. Johnson suggests that any heavy drinker might do well to give himself a test to determine whether or not he is an alcoholic. It only requires that the drinker declare twice a year an alcohol holiday of not less than a week. If he can do this without feeling withdrawal symptoms and martyrdom, and with no obsessive desire to return to drinking when the test period is over, alcoholism is not yet present.

Are some drinks less intoxicating than others?

Bloody marys and screwdrivers may be less so than most other mixed drinks. Both the bloody mary with its tomato juice and the screwdriver with its orange juice are high in fructose, a type of sugar found in many fruits.

In one recent study in Boston, twelve male alcoholic volunteers were given fructose injections at the same time they were drinking bourbon. They were not nearly as intoxicated as others who did not receive the injections. Several men who got the fructose injections claimed somebody had watered their bourbon.

Fructose was actually found to lower alcohol levels in the blood by 43 percent, usually within fifteen minutes. It may do so by speeding breakdown of alcohol. In another study, in which subjects drank fructose along with their alcohol, blood alcohol levels also fell.

Does any treatment for alcoholism work?

Alcoholism has to be looked upon as a chronic illness. The goal of all current treatment is total abstinence because, with rare exceptions, just one drink can start the whole cycle over again. Treatment includes psychotherapy, medication, and Alcoholics Anonymous.

An alcoholic can be helped over the withdrawal process with drugs such as chlordiazepoxide (Librium), magnesium sulfate, and vitamin B complex. Psychiatric help—sometimes even relatively short-term help—may be valuable. For some patients, a drug such as disulfiram (Antabuse) may be prescribed; it produces distinctly unpleasant effects only when alcohol is taken.

Alcoholics Anonymous is of prime importance. For those who can and will accept it, it may be the only form of treatment required.

What makes AA tick?

It's interesting to try to figure out why it has been more successful than doctors, sociologists, clergymen, or anybody else who has ever tried to work with alcoholics. That's been true since AA began in 1934.

Its members are dedicated, and extremely varied. Many have simple jobs, little education, and modest means, but they mingle well with highly educated professionals, men of genius and fame, and the very wealthy. The common ground is that each member has a story of heartbreak because of alcoholism, heartbreak in terms of career or family problems.

The chief medical officer for a major industrial firm, who has seen AA's results with all kinds of employees under his medical supervision, suggests that an alcoholic facing a non-alcoholic trying to help him (however kind and understanding the would-be helper is) feels a sense of guilt, inferiority, or plain discomfort. Because it's an unpleasant feeling, the alcoholic brushes off treatment one way or another.

But when he joins an AA group at a meeting, he feels he belongs. All members are on the same level; there is no condescension, all is friendly, pleasant, easygoing. At one time or another, an AA group hears the story of each individual member.

It comforts the teller to unload his story; it comforts the listener who can compare his own experience with that of the teller.

Moreover, AA becomes a way of life. Members devote several evenings a week to it, helping others after they themselves have overcome their alcoholism. They love it, which is not really startling since it's the rare person who doesn't like the satisfaction of helping others.

Alcoholism is a way of life that becomes unbearable eventually. Treatment is largely directed at helping the victim find a new way of life. AA does this remarkably well.

With all of modern research, hasn't anybody found a cure for hangover?

There is no cure, but some methods may speed relief from hangover. The throbbing head pain from alcohol's dilation of blood vessels in the head can be alleviated by medications containing caffeine and ergotamine, the same kind of medication used for migraine headaches. Caffeine in black coffee also helps constrict the blood vessels and end the headache.

Alcohol dehydrates the body, but drinking water alone to assuage that may increase nausea; several cups of salted beef broth at intervals will replace water and minerals and reduce nausea. Alcohol ordinarily is broken down by the body at a constant rate; fructose helps the body burn it up faster. Fructose is found in honey, ripe fruits, vegetables, and extracts such as tomato juice.

Some English physicians lately have found that antihistamines —the medications often used for allergies—may be of some help in getting rid of hangovers.

Does sleep have anything to do with longevity?

Theories that good sleep can forestall aging are based on the idea that toxic materials are formed daily in the body as the result of activity, stress, and anxiety, and that profound, untroubled sleep gets rid of them. But such sleep becomes rarer with age; the theories have argued that since the sleep of the aged is shallow and easily broken, toxins are less adequately eliminated and this may account at least in part for the physical changes of aging. But the theories are just that—not established fact.

Some investigators argue that if toxins build up by day and good sleep eliminates them by night, then every healthy youth and young adult ought to leap out of bed in the morning in a state of exuberance after a good night's sleep—but that doesn't always happen.

But sleep is essential?

Yes. Without it, we feel not only physically fatigued but also emotionally drained. The longest a person can go without sleep, studies have shown, is about ten days. Volunteers who have been deprived of sleep for such extensive periods have found the experience a torture. Even after only sixty-five hours without sleep, one volunteer was discovered in a washroom, frantically trying to wash "cobwebs" off his face, convinced he was covered with them.

How much sleep is really necessary?

It's generally assumed that eight hours of sleep is the norm. But scientific studies show a wide range of sleep requirements. A study in Scotland showed that 8 percent of a large sample needed five hours maximum, and some got along with less. Fifteen percent needed five to six hours, and the large bulk of people needed seven to eight hours. But 13 percent required nine to ten hours, and a few needed even more than ten. Even among infants there are marked differences. The assumption has been that every newborn spends about twenty hours of the day asleep, but studies show a range from ten to twenty-three.

Any accounting for the need variations?

There have been suggestions that body type may be involved, that the endomorph—the soft, fat type of person—sleeps easily and a lot; the ectomorph—sensitive and fragile—is prone to insomnia. But no definite studies support this idea.

However, scientists wouldn't be at all surprised if there were a built-in genetically determined predisposition for the amount of sleep one needs. Although training and environment *are* factors in sleep habits as they are in eating and other habits, Dr. Julius Segal of the National Institute of Mental Health observes: "The old phrase, 'born that way,' referring to genetic inheritance, seems increasingly relevant here. That is, the patterns of sleep that many people exhibit or complain about are apparent from earliest childhood. Many parents who are very upset about a child's sleep patterns ought best to make peace with the fact that those patterns came with the child and are not all that easy to change."

How can one find out how many hours of sleep he really needs?

One way is to pick some period when you're relatively free of stress. A vacation period may be a good time. Go to bed at the same time each night for a period of two to three weeks, and get up in the morning without help from an alarm clock. The average length of nightly sleep during a period like that is probably close to what is normal for you.

Are there best hours for sleeping?

No one set of hours is best for everybody. Some people like to retire late and get up late; others prefer going to bed early and getting up early. Each to his own. The old idea that one hour of sleep before midnight is worth two hours after midnight is a myth.

What happens in the body during sleep?

A lot of the old notions about sleep have been upset by very recent studies in sleep laboratories using delicate equipment to detect and amplify brain currents, monitor eye movements, and record pulse rate, breathing rate, body movements, and muscle tensions.

Once it was thought that sleep was a state of complete oblivion. Now it's known that sleep is a matter of rhythmic cycles.

As you close your eyes in preparation for sleep, body temperature begins to fall and brain waves show what is called alpha rhythm, a frequency of about nine to thirteen cycles per second. You are still awake but beginning to move into sleep. In stage I sleep, the pulse slows, muscles relax, and brain waves slow to four to six cycles per second; this is light sleep.

In stage II, medium-deep sleep, brain waves grow larger and slower. After about thirty minutes you move into stage III, and the waves slow still more. Deepest sleep, stage IV, comes next; it lasts only about twenty minutes, whereupon you begin to move into lighter sleep again. As you do, you may make some movement, turn in bed, and almost, but not quite, reach the conscious level. Now your eyes begin to move under the closed lids in much the same fashion as when you watch a movie. At this point you are dreaming, and if you were to be awakened at this point, you would recall the dream very clearly. After about ten minutes of this rapid eye movement (REM), or dreaming sleep, you start the whole cycle all over again. Each cycle takes about ninety minutes.

One thing is clear: everyone needs to dream. Exactly why is still something of a mystery. But when investigators have wakened subjects every time they entered REM sleep, but let them sleep at other times, the subjects showed impaired physical and psychological functioning.

We now know that nobody sleeps through the night "like a log." Nor does sleep become increasingly deeper through the night; it keeps shifting in the ninety-minute cycles.

Do we know what purpose dreaming serves?

One theory suggested by a distinguished British psychologist, Dr. Christopher Evans, holds that dreaming is a surface manifestation of a complex brain process in which bits of information gathered during the day are moved from short-term to long-term memory circuits. Somewhat like a computer, Evans believes, the brain has to go "off-line," disconnecting itself from controls, before it can reshuffle the information. If it didn't, if the reshuffling went on while the brain was awake, what we experience during sleep as gentle dreams might well become hallucinations. In fact, Evans says, many nightmares occur when the brain accidentally comes "on-line" during the transfer process.

Do sleep habits reflect personality traits?

So it seems, from studies made by Dr. Ernest Hartmann, director of the sleep laboratory of Boston State Hospital. Hartmann and his colleagues selected twenty-nine volunteers, some who habitually slept less than six hours and others who habitually slept more than eight. The volunteers were required to sleep eight nights at the sleep laboratory, during which they underwent a variety of tests.

Overall, the people who slept less were more socially adept and dominant in relationships with others. Their vocations included engineering, business, carpentry, and contracting. They tended to be comformists, establishment-oriented in job preference and opinions. They kept busy, and tended to avoid psychological problems rather than face them.

The people who slept more had a greater variety of professions and interests. Many held responsible jobs, some were artists, a few were described as hippies. They were less conformist, and some were very creative. But many were shy, some were mildly depressed, and some appeared anxious. Most were somewhat inhibited sexually.

Hartmann noted during the experiment that the people who slept more had about twice as much REM, or dream sleep, as the ones who slept less. Conceivably, he thinks, they may need to sleep longer and dream more in order to use the greater dream time to resolve psychic problems.

Does everybody suffer from occasional insomnia?

Very likely, since all of us experience unusual stresses at one time or another. Such stresses may make it more difficult to fall asleep or stay asleep.

Is there such a thing as imaginary insomnia?

Apparently there is. Many people believe, quite honestly, that sometimes they get no sleep at all. But laboratory studies have shown how easy it is to be misled.

For one thing, it can be difficult to judge one's own sleep. In one study, people claiming they didn't sleep at all agreed to press a signal button whenever, during the night in the laboratory, they heard a buzzer sound. They were monitored by electro-encephalogram and in every case brain waves showed sleep. Microphones also picked up gentle snoring. Although the buzzer was sounded several times, no button was pressed in reply. Yet in the morning the subjects protested that they hadn't slept at all. Some dream-recall studies suggest that, for some people, dreams tend to fuse with reality. Upon being wakened after a period of REM sleep, such people often claim they have been thinking rather than dreaming.

Dr. Julius Segal of the National Institute of Mental Health tells of a psychologist who volunteered to be a subject in a sleep study. When he woke the next morning, exhausted, he apologized to the research team for giving them so little of his sleep to analyze. But his colleagues laughed, assured him that few volunteers had done as much sleeping as he had. In six good hours of sleep, however, there had been many points at which brain-wave recordings indicated the waking alpha rhythm, suggesting he was at the edge of near-awakening. These moments of near-awakening, Segal thinks, may have fused in his mind, leaving him convinced he had been continuously on the borderline of waking.

With all the new insights into sleep, are there more
effective ways now to combat insomnia?

There are. It's clear now that a lot of people get trapped into the habit of using sleeping pills because they fear a temporary period of insomnia. A sensible thing to do in such a period, many physicians suggest, is not to just lie sleepless in bed and get agitated about it. Get up, balance your checkbook, read a book, or listen to music. If you occupy yourself rather than fight for sleep, then go back to bed after half an hour or an hour, you'll probably be drowsy again.

At one medical center a considerable amount of sleep research has been done with severe insomniacs. The physician-investigators encourage them to gradually increase activity and exercise levels during the day but not to be active near bedtime hours. They've found that exercise some hours before sleep increases stage IV sleep, but exercise just prior to bedtime has an exciting effect.

Patients are also instructed to establish a regular hour for retiring but not to remain in bed if they don't fall asleep. They are also urged to maintain relaxing mental attitudes just before bedtime, avoiding any complex mental activity.

Sometimes these suggestions alone work. When they don't, drugs are prescribed according to a specific sleep difficulty. For difficulty in falling asleep, a drug such as flurazepam is prescribed. Difficulty in staying asleep often indicates mental depression; for such patients, in addition to flurazepam at bedtime, antidepressant medication for use during the day is prescribed.

Do drugs allow normal sleep?

Some more so than others. Actually, with prolonged use, some sleeping pills cause trouble because they inhibit the dream stage of sleep. People kept from dreaming tend to become irritable and anxious. An added danger is that after using such pills for an extended period, horrible nightmares may be experienced when the pills are discontinued; it's as if the body is trying to make up for the lost dreams. The nightmares may make the victims go back to pill taking.

If you need drugs to help you over a period of severe insomnia, the safest bet is to have a physician prescribe a suitable one for you rather than to use someone else's prescription drug or a nonprescription drug.

What about the folk remedies for insomnia?

It's hardly a cure, but research indicates that warm milk does in fact contain the amino acid tryptophan, which has been shown to have a sedative effect.

Some people like to take a drink before bedtime to relieve insomnia. Since alcohol is a depressant, it can produce drowsiness. But responses differ, and alcohol makes some people irritable or stimulated. Excessive alcohol, like some sleeping pills, reduces dream sleep, and that's not desirable.

Is sleep therapy—prolonged sleep—effective for physical disorders?

Sleep treatment is in use in the Soviet Union, but it hasn't come into wide use in the United States. Dr. Leon Marder of the University of Southern California School of Medicine has done some work with sleep therapy and believes that it has value.

Marder demonstrated the powers of sleep in a research project in which a dozen patients suffering from a variety of ailments, including ulcers, migraine, high blood pressure, and gastrointestinal disorders, recovered after two weeks of prolonged sleep. Drugs kept the patients asleep for eighteen to twenty hours a day. They awakened for meals, light exercise, and informal psychiatric consultations. During the third week, they were gradually returned to normal sleeping habits, without use of drugs. In the nearly two years since then, they have had no recurrence of symptoms.

The patients previously had failed to respond to medication and psychotherapy. Without exception, they had emotional problems. Because they were ill emotionally and physically, they weren't getting proper sleep, and because they weren't getting proper sleep, Marder believes, they were irritable, defeated, less able to deal with their problems. Rested and refreshed after sleep therapy, they were able, according to Marder, to handle their emotional problems without any help from attending psychiatrists.

What does relaxation have to do with longevity?

No definitive statistical studies show a neat relationship between relaxation and longevity. But that's just as true for sleep.

Relaxation—periods of respite during the day and the week, and of vacation one or more times a year—is not much less, if at all less, important than sleep for health, productivity, overall satisfaction, and pleasure with work and family, all of which count in the longevity picture. Sleep is needed to overcome fatigue; so is relaxation.

A surprising number of people believe that time off is time wasted. They discount leisure, which is a big mistake. (See the discussion of "workaholics" in chapter 7.)

One distinguished physician, recently queried about modern stresses and strains, observed, "If more of us were concerned with the art of living than with the quest for longevity, we'd live more happily and productively, and perhaps longer, too." Relaxation is part of the art of living.

Any evidence of specific values of relaxation?

As many physicians tell it, it's hard to find among people who know how to relax any potential nervous breakdown victims. People who can relax seem to have a large degree of protection against such ailments as irritable bowel, heartburn, migraine, ulcerative colitis, and other serious disorders. Before modern medicines were available, relaxation was a major element in arresting and curing tuberculosis. It still is very much part of the treatment for heart disease patients.

Relaxation also increases working productivity. There have been many studies showing that when working time is shortened, hourly productivity tends to go up, while lengthening working time has the opposite effect. It's been found that in addition to cutting down productivity per hour, overtime work is often accompanied by increased absences due to illness and accidents.

To be sure, these investigations have been carried out in factories and have covered physical work. Studies of the relationship between mental productivity and working hours are needed. But there is no reason to suppose that overwork does not impair mental performance when we know that relaxation—change of scene and change of pace—can improve it.

Actually, studies in neurophysiology provide a better understanding of the importance of rest and relaxation. Investigators have been able to locate specific brain structures in animals, stimulate them with small electrical currents, and show that certain brain structures have an inhibitory effect, while others constitute an activating system.

Mood and ability to perform at any given time depend on the degree of activity of the two systems. When the inhibitory system is dominant, the individual is in a state of fatigue. When the activating system is dominant, he is ready to increase performance.

The existence of the two systems helps to explain some previously puzzling phenomena. For example, everyone has had the experience of feeling physically or mentally fatigued but when something unexpected happens—maybe it's good news or bad, or a sudden inspiration—the fatigue disappears. What has happened is that the activating system has been stimulated by the unexpected and has attained dominance over the inhibitory system.

Even after a good night's sleep and just a few hours of work, not enough to produce physical fatigue, we may become mentally fatigued and bored if the surroundings are monotonous and the job is dull. Then the activating system is dampened and the inhibitory one becomes dominant.

Monotony involves sameness. And even the most thought-provoking, challenging work can become monotonous if it goes on day after day, or even hour after hour, without change of pace.

"Time out is not time lost," one physician puts it. Properly used, relaxation restores stamina and patience, renews good attitude toward a job, and helps the sense of humor. The dividends have a favorable influence upon a man's physical health, which is indispensable to his effectiveness and productivity.

What's the best way to relax from day to day?

There isn't one best way. A long time ago, the distinguished physician Sir William Osler put it this way: "No man is really happy or safe without a hobby, and it makes precious little difference what the outside interest may be—botany, beetles, or butterflies; roses, tulips, or irises; fishing, mountaineering, or antiquities—anything will do so long as he straddles a hobby and rides it hard."

In addition to hobbies during nonworking hours, there are opportunities during the day to get a change of pace. It's possible for some to spend part of a lunch hour exercising at a gym or athletic club. There may be opportunity at lunchtime only for a walk, which can be relaxing. For the sedentary worker especially, a sport or other physical activity can give beneficial relaxation.

Presumably, vacations are beneficial to health?

They can be and should be, but the value of a vacation depends on many things.

The ancient Hebrew lawgivers decreed that every seventh year the land should be left uncultivated so it could renew itself. In the Middle Ages, the Christian fathers invented the sabbatical, a layoff every seventh year. If you can't have a sabbatical, you can at least sample the balm on a vacation. Says the chairman of the board of one of the country's biggest corporations: "We regard the rest period as a vital component of a year's total work situation, and I constantly remind our people that they are not scoring points with the corporation by refusing to take their vacations."

14

Hidden
Problems

What are the hidden problems?

They are three diseases—hypertension or high blood pressure, diabetes, and gout—that are somewhat unique. They can be disturbing in themselves; they can also exist without giving away their presence. They are significant contributory factors in the greatest killer—coronary heart disease. All three are far more common than popularly supposed. And all three can, if detected, be treated effectively.

What, in fact, is blood pressure? And when is it considered high?

Blood pressure is simply a force against the walls of arteries. Each time the heart beats and pumps blood into the arteries, the pressure increases; in the interval between beats, the pressure goes down. When a physician measures pressure, he makes two readings and writes them in the form of a fraction—for example, 130/80. The first and larger figure is the systolic pressure (when the heart pumps); the second is the diastolic pressure (when the heart rests).

It's usual for blood pressure to fluctuate, decreasing during sleep and rest, increasing during physical exertion or emotional excitement. And there is a considerable range of normal. At rest a systolic pressure in the 100-to-140 range and a diastolic in the 60-to-90 range is considered normal. A single reading above 140/90 does not necessarily mean abnormal pressure. But when there is continuous elevation, a person is considered to have hypertension.

How common is hypertension?

By the very lowest estimate, at least one of every ten people in this country—20 million—is hypertensive. Some studies suggest a far higher incidence. According to one survey of a sample of people supposed to be representative of the total population, the incidence is 29 percent. Of those taking part in another nationwide survey, 33.9 percent had elevated blood pressure. At Johns Hopkins Medical School in Baltimore, 1,139 medical students were first examined at a mean age of twenty-three, then followed for eight to twenty-two years; in that period 42.4 percent developed hypertension.

People with hypertension can be rich, poor, white, black, young, and old. The common notion that the disease affects mostly the elderly is not true. It affects the middle-aged, the young adults, even children. According to a recent study, hypertensive tendencies can be detected in the offspring of hypertensive parents even as early as the age of two.

What are the symptoms of hypertension?

There may be none at all. The disease is stealthy. Even when it does produce some symptoms—headaches, dizziness, fatigue, or weakness—they may not be recognized for what they are, since they are common to many other disorders. Most cases of hypertension are not recognized by the people who have the disease; the condition is uncovered during medical examinations. When, for example, employees at one large Michigan industrial plant were screened for hypertension, 919 were found to have it—but 78 percent of them had no idea that they had it. You can pretty well count on it: If you have hypertension, the chances are you won't know you have it unless you're told so by a physician.

Just how great a danger is hypertension?

Increasing evidence shows that, if left untreated, hypertension is one of the gravest of diseases. It is a major factor in heart attacks and also in strokes and potentially fatal kidney disease.

Almost forty years ago one physician noted that 60 percent of his patients with heart attacks had elevated pressure. In a 1948 survey of young soldiers, there were more than four times as many coronary deaths among those with elevated pressure as among those with normal pressure. More recently, the Framingham study has shown a far greater risk of coronary disease among hypertensives—a threefold increase in the risk, for example, among men forty to fifty-five years of age.

Investigators of the Health Insurance Plan of Greater New York recently found that among men who had hypertension before a first heart attack, the number dead within one month after the attack was more than twice that of men with normal pressure who had a first heart attack. Moreover, compared with men with normal pressure who survive a first attack, hypertensive men who survive have twice the risk of recurrence and more than five times the risk of death from heart trouble during the next four and a half years.

What is the effect of hypertension on stroke and kidney disease?

The risk of stroke in the Framingham study has been found to be five times as high among people with even just moderately elevated pressure levels (160/95) as among normal people. "Not only is high blood pressure the major cause of stroke in young people," says Dr. Richard E. Lee, physician-in-charge of the New York Hospital's high blood pressure clinic, "but those who don't die of stroke may die of kidney disease."

Dr. Oglesby Paul, former American Heart Association president and now Professor of Medicine at Northwestern University, declares, "It is not too much to say that the diagnosis, study, and treatment of mild hypertension in young and middle-aged adults constitutes one of our greatest health challenges today."

How does high blood pressure exert its effects?

Excessive pressure burdens the heart, which must pump harder against that pressure. The burden is constant, and after a time the heart may enlarge as a result. But it's not a healthy enlargement (like that of the athlete's heart) and often abnormalities of heartbeat result. Each year about 50,000 Americans die from this problem, which is called hypertensive heart disease.

Bad as that is, it is overshadowed by coronary heart disease, which leads to heart attacks. Over a period of years, elevated pressure strains artery walls and may damage them. In a way, it's like forcing water through a garden hose at pressures higher than the hose is designed to take; eventually, the hose will be damaged.

The artery walls are injured; cholesterol and other fatty materials circulating in the blood may then nest in the damaged areas. Heightened pressure may even force the fats into the artery walls. The vessels then narrow and have reduced capacity for carrying blood. Sometimes a vessel may become completely blocked; if the vessel is a coronary artery feeding the heart, a heart attack may well follow. If the narrowed vessel is an artery feeding the brain, a stroke may follow. Or if the narrowed vessel feeds a kidney, kidney trouble will result.

What causes elevated pressure?

In only 10 to 15 percent of cases can some definite physical cause be found. It may be a narrowing (coarctation) of the aorta, the great artery that carries blood from the heart; this is curable by an operation that eliminates the narrowing. An adrenal gland tumor (pheochromocytoma) is usually benign, but it produces large quantities of hormones that raise blood pressure; it, too, is curable by surgery. Obstruction to normal blood flow in a kidney artery may lead to elevated pressure; it can be cured by the insertion of a synthetic tube to bypass the obstruction.

But in 85 to 90 percent of cases, there is no apparent physical cause for hypertension. This is what is known as essential hypertension, which simply means that the cause is unknown.

How is essential hypertension treated?

In some mild cases nothing more than weight reduction may be needed. Elevated pressure often is associated with excess weight and tends to be reduced when the overweight person reduces. If the pressure is only mildly elevated, it may fall to normal levels.

Excessive salt in the diet may raise pressure. Experiments have established that laboratory animals placed on high-salt diets develop hypertension and die early. Some patients, especially those with milder degrees of hypertension, benefit by salt reduction. In fact, until not many years ago, before effective drug therapy was available, severe salt restriction was a mainstay of treatment.

Many different drugs are now available to treat hypertension.

Diuretic drugs increase the body's excretion of salt so that a severely salt-restricted and tasteless diet no longer is required.

Certain mild drugs act as calmatives in the central nervous system, reducing the flow of exciting impulses that can raise blood pressure. Certain other drugs, from the relatively mild to the extremely potent, lower pressure by blocking certain nerve pathways or by relaxing tiny blood vessels involved in raising pressure. The physician can choose a drug likely to be suitable, try it, combine it with another when necessary, and adjust dosage until he finds the drug or combination of drugs that can control pressure effectively and produce minimal or no side effects.

Is treatment always effective?

In the overwhelming majority of cases treatment is effective, even for a most severe form, called malignant hypertension, which once progressed so rapidly that it was often fatal within a year after being diagnosed.

The effectiveness of treatment makes neglect of hypertension all the more tragic. According to Dr. Jeremiah Stamler of the Chicago Health Research Foundation, approximately half the hypertensive people in the country are undetected, "half of those that are detected go untreated, and only about half of those receiving treatment have had their blood pressures brought down to levels of less than 90 diastolic and less than 140 systolic."

Why the neglect?

It is often difficult to get people to take pressure elevation seriously. Most have no symptoms with their hypertension. For early diagnosis there must be regular checkups, and many people don't get regular checkups.

But even many who get checkups and are diagnosed as having hypertension start treatment, only to give it up quickly because they have no symptoms. They find it hard to believe that anything can be wrong if they feel well.

In one special program carried out in Baldwin County, Georgia, public health nurses were sent to make house-to-house calls on a large sample of the population, some 3,000 persons. They found 630 with high blood pressure. Of these, 45 percent had had no idea they had hypertension. Even among the 347 who knew they had it, there was neglect. Most had stopped taking their medicine within three months. After tabulating all the data from the study, Dr. Joseph A. Wilber, director of the Georgia Public Health Department's Cardiovascular Control Service, concluded that, all told, only about 14 percent of the hypertensive cases were being adequately treated.

Another problem has been that many physicians have had a lukewarm or antipathetic attitude about treatment in many cases. Not for the very severe cases. For them, treatment has been regarded as absolutely essential. For people with malignant hypertension, treatment has been accepted as lifesaving.

But for a long time there was considerable doubt about the value of treating moderate and mild hypertension. What was needed was a clear scientific evaluation of just how much good is done when mild and moderate hypertension are controlled. Now that evaluation is available.

How much good is accomplished by bringing down mild and moderate elevations?

A tremendous amount of good. Beginning in 1963, a Veterans Administration Cooperative Study Group, chaired by Dr. Edward D. Freis of Washington, D.C., undertook a long-term study. Eighteen VA hospitals across the country participated.

First, the group studied effects of treatment in patients with moderate hypertension—those with 115 to 129 diastolic pressures, as opposed to a normal upper limit of 90. They ranged upward in age from thirty. Some got active treatment with antihypertensive medication; some, for comparison, got placebo (inactive) pills. There were no deaths among the actively treated patients; there were four deaths among the others. There were twenty-seven serious incidents—heart attacks, strokes, congestive heart failure—among the placebo patients, but only two such incidents among the treated. The study was stopped earlier than planned in the placebo group so they could be switched to active treatment to reduce their risk.

More recently, the study group investigated treatment value in patients with mild hypertension—with diastolic pressures in the range of only 90 to 104, just barely above the upper limit for normal. The study, lasting more than five years, covered 380 men. Again there were two groups, actively treated and placebo. The results left no room for doubt: among the treated men, the heart attack and stroke risk was cut by two-thirds. Moreover, twenty of the men in the placebo group went on to develop severe hypertension; none of the treated men did. As Dr. Freis and his colleagues have noted: "Certain complications such as congestive heart failure, hypertensive neuroretinopathy [an eye complication], strokes, and kidney deterioration were reduced or essentially eleminated in the treated patients. In addition, treatment prevented elevation of diastolic blood pressure to levels where the risk of developing complications is greatly increased."

The VA studies confirmed some smaller but equally impressive studies made in England. One involved ten hypertensive men without symptoms who were treated. None had any complications over a period of up to six years, while among twelve other men not receiving treatment, four had strokes, one had a heart attack, and two developed heart failure. In another English study, patients who already had had a stroke were divided into treated and untreated groups. Of the forty-two untreated for hypertension, only 66 percent were alive at the end of five years; of the thirty-nine treated, 90 percent were alive.

Do doctors now take hypertension seriously?

More doctors now believe strongly in treating even mild hypertension. The ideal is to bring blood pressure to normal levels and keep it there. Many physicians find that it is helpful for patients to take their own pressure readings at home. The home measurements often give a truer picture of the blood pressure than those in the doctor's office; there is no anxiety connected with home measurements. And they simplify treatment, by making fewer visits to the physician necessary.

Can hypertension affect intellect?

An added reason—if one were needed—for watching and keeping blood pressure under control comes from a recent study suggesting that the decline in mental abilities in older people may often have less to do with aging than with elevated pressure.

Dr. Carl Eisdorfer and Dr. Frances Wilkie of Duke University's Center for the Study of Aging and Human Development observed a group of men and women in their sixties over a ten-year period. At the start, the subjects were divided into groups on the basis of whether blood pressure was elevated or not. Every 2.5 years, each patient got a thorough physical examination plus a complete battery of psychological and intelligence tests.

Among those whose blood pressure was normal, there was no intellectual change even at the end of ten years; among those with high blood pressure, test scores fell almost ten points.

Do very young people with pressure elevations really run much of a risk?

At Duke University Medical Center Dr. Siegfried Heyden and a medical team were able to trace thirty teen-agers who, seven years before, had been found to have blood pressure elevations, often mild. They had had no treatment. Two had already died of stroke; one had hypertensive heart disease; three had developed brain and heart symptoms; five others were as yet without symptoms, but they had markedly elevated pressures.

A major factor in those who develop increasingly severe hypertension and complications seems to be weight gain. The Duke physicians suggest that a weight-gaining adolescent who has even mild pressure elevation should be treated with a weight-reduction program as well as antihypertensive medication.

Can oral contraceptives cause hypertension?

In some women hypertension does accompany the use of the Pill. How often this occurs is not known. In one recent study a rise in blood pressure was found in eleven of sixty-two women using oral contraceptives. The pressure may rise weeks to months after starting the Pill and usually falls within four weeks after use is discontinued. An editorial in the *Journal of the American Medical Association* recently called the attention of physicians to "the need for occasionally measuring the blood pressure of every patient taking the Pill."

What exactly should one do about the possibility of having hypertension?

If you suspect you have it, or if you've been told in the past that you had a mild or borderline elevation and have done nothing about it, it would be wise to see your physician now, find out what the pressure currently is, and get his advice on bringing it down if it is elevated.

If hypertension has never been diagnosed, recognize that no one is immune and that pressure can go up at any time without warning symptoms. A pressure measurement should be part of every medical checkup. If, by any chance, your physician doesn't include it in your checkups, insist that he do so or find a physician who does it. Most physicians do so routinely.

What's the importance of diabetes?

Like hypertension, it's a disorder that almost every heart disease expert believes accelerates the course of coronary atherosclerosis. Like hypertension, it is much more common than often is supposed. Although it is very often easily treatable, it is often allowed to go undetected and untreated. Of an estimated 4.4

million diabetics in the country, 1.6 million are currently undiagnosed.

Why is diabetes so often undiagnosed?

Diabetes is a sneaky disease. It doesn't signal its presence with unmistakable pain or produce any clear-cut early warning signs. Typically, in early stages, many victims simply feel somewhat listless and run-down; they seek no medical aid.

The early Greeks gave diabetes its name. The word means "siphon" in Greek. More than a 1,000 years ago a Greek physician wrote of it as "a disease in which the flesh melts away, is siphoned off in the urine." This definition often holds true in late stages, if the disease is uncontrolled.

What's involved in diabetes?

At the heart of the disease is a failure to utilize carbohydrates properly. The body is especially dependent upon one carbohydrate, a sugar called glucose, which is derived from food. Normally a fairly constant level of glucose is maintained in the blood to provide a source of energy for body functions. Insulin, a hormone produced by the pancreas, regulates the level of sugar in the blood and also promotes its use by body tissues.

Diabetes results from lack of insulin or from inability of insulin to act effectively. In the diabetic condition glucose cannot be used properly, accumulates in the blood, and then spills over through the kidneys into the urine to be excreted. The siphoning off of glucose leads to excessive urination, one major symptom of fairly well-advanced diabetes, and to thirst, another symptom.

Diabetes also leads to tissue starvation. In uncontrolled diabetes the body is unable to utilize sugar and so it eventually scavenges, attacking its own cells to get nutrition, and weight loss and debility follow. In its attempts to get enough energy, the body also resorts to excessive breakdown of fats, which produces toxic substances called ketone bodies, or ketoacids. These enter the blood and can cause diabetic acidosis, coma, and death.

Daily insulin injections can control diabetes. But until 1921, when insulin was isolated, diabetes patients were doomed to just such a terrible progression. Previously only dietary restrictions were known to help, and often these failed. The best a newly discovered diabetic could hope for was five to ten years of life, most of them miserable years.

In the mid-fifties oral antidiabetes drugs were developed. Their use soon helped to confirm what some physicians had suspected—diabetes exists in more than one form. The oral drugs confirmed this suspicion because they helped many adults but had little value for child diabetics. Children with diabetes had to have injections of insulin.

In 1962 came another development which changed the picture of diabetes. There long had been tests to measure sugar in the blood. Now came a test to measure insulin in the blood. The test showed that most diabetics actually had no insulin deficiency; in fact, they had excess amounts of insulin as well as sugar in the blood. These were the diabetics, some 80 percent of the total number, who had developed the disease in adulthood.

Diabetes is now divided into two main types: growth-onset diabetes, which appears before age fifteen, and is characterized by little or no ability to produce insulin; and maturity-onset diabetes, which develops later in life, with more than adequate production of insulin but inability to use the insulin effectively.

Who gets diabetes?

Anybody can, with or without a history of the disorder in the family. But it does tend to run in families. A child of two diabetics has a 100 percent likelihood of getting diabetes if he or she lives long enough. And the child of one diabetic parent has a 50 percent chance.

The familial incidence becomes increasingly strong. Women who have had diabetes since childhood today have high rates of fertility in contrast to the pre-insulin era, when pregnancy among uncontrolled diabetics was rare and often fatal. Moreover, modern drugs have reduced the death toll from infectious diseases so people live longer, and the number of diabetics grows because the chance of getting diabetes increases with age.

In addition to the more than 4 million diagnosed and undiagnosed diabetics, there appears to be an even greater total of those who are progressing into diabetes. In one large Public Health Service screening program, 10 percent of an unselected adult population proved positive.

A few years ago, when Chicago hospitals began to make it a rule to test all patients for diabetes no matter what the reason for their hospitalization, they uncovered large numbers with the disease. At one hospital 6 percent of newly admitted patients were found to have diabetes without knowing it. In another hospital 27 percent of patients showed borderline responses to testing, indicating they had or were on the verge of having diabetes.

A few years ago, to help get a statewide diabetes detection program under way, 265 New Hampshire legislators took diabetes tests themselves. Eighty-four of them—one in five—were astounded to learn that they had diabetes.

Some authorities estimate that 25 percent of Americans either are or may become diabetic. Six percent inherit the trait from both parents and are diabetic. Nineteen percent inherit from one parent; they are carriers of the disease and many will develop it as they age.

On top of this has come the recognition that diabetes is an "iceberg" disease." Sugar in the blood is only the tip of the iceberg. Other manifestations, particularly the influence of diabetes in heart disease, are of great significance.

How does diabetes affect the heart?

The biggest single cause of death among diabetics is coronary heart disease. As many as 77 percent of deaths in diabetics are due to blood vessel diseases of one kind or another. At the Joslin Clinic, a famed diabetes research and treatment center, 46.5 percent of deaths in diabetics have been caused by coronary heart disease. Autopsy studies of diabetics have shown coronary heart disease present in 75 percent to 98 percent.

To check on various factors influencing health, researchers in Tecumseh, Michigan persuaded 8,600 Tecumseh residents, nine-tenths of the community, to undergo blood and urine tests, electrocardiograms, and complete physical exams. They were hardly surprised to find a high frequency of coronary disease among the diabetics in the population. For the first time on record, they found that people with heart disease tended to have diabetes. It appeared that many with coronary disease could be mild diabetics in whom the coronary problem either came before or overshadowed the sugar-handling abnormality.

Significantly, then, a high sugar level in the blood could be an important factor in predicting the possibility of heart disease, even of heart attack.

Such factors as excess cholesterol in the blood, high blood pressure, and obesity, all linked to coronary heart disease, are present in diabetes. Researchers have found that cholesterol levels tend to be higher in diabetics than in people without diabetes, that hypertension is nearly twice as frequent, and that four of every five newly discovered diabetics either are or have been fatter than they should be.

Dr. Glen McDonald of the Public Health Service has observed: "We have obesity, hypertension, and abnormal blood levels of cholesterol and sugar in both diabetes and heart disease. We have known for some time that most diabetics will eventually die of cardiovascular disease. And from the time of the Tecumseh study, it began to be apparent that a great many patients with heart disease were also showing abnormalities of carbohydrate metabolism.

"Since then, investigators have looked to determine how these abnormalities might relate to diabetes. In one such study, researchers performed tests on ninety-five patients with arteriosclerosis—all supposed to be nondiabetic. In 46 percent test results were in the diabetic range. These investigators also cited a study in Sweden which showed that the prevalence of diabetes was five times higher in cases of coronary thrombosis than in the general population.

"What can we conclude from all these correlations? We must accept the conclusion that diabetes is heavily implicated in the leading cause of death—heart disease. These diseases are related diseases. Those who have been singled out through scientific investigation as high-risk people for heart disease are the same people we know to be high-risk people for diabetes. We must find these people, these early or so-called mild diabetics. And we must find them a lot earlier than we have been finding them up to now."

What exactly is the score on weight and diabetes?

There is an interesting new view today. It has long been accepted that excess weight is a factor in triggering diabetes. Now some investigators believe that excess weight may be part of the diabetes, a kind of early indication of the disease, in some cases.

In as many as 85 percent of people who develop diabetes in adulthood, obesity is present. Is the obesity that precedes the diabetes, sometimes by many years, a result of the same defect that later produces the impairment of carbohydrate handling? Some think so.

At one recent conference, a group of investigators from Hahnemann Medical College in Philadelphia reported testing 238 obese people for diabetes. Six clearly had diabetes. Ninety-one others had sugar levels identifying them as latent diabetics. Moreover, 104 others had abnormally low blood sugar levels and abnormally high insulin levels. They had what is called reactive hypoglycemia (low blood sugar), which has been regarded by some researchers in the past as a possible early sign of diabetes. Now, the Hahnemann physicians suggest, the finding of reactive hypoglycemia in obese patients supports the idea that obesity represents a stage in the early development of diabetes. As they see it, an obese individual may have an unduly sensitive pancreas, which releases more insulin than normal in response to food intake. The excess insulin lowers blood sugar beyond normal. This increases appetite. And there may then be a vicious cycle resulting in obesity.

Dr. W. J. H. Butterfield of Guys Hospital Medical School, London, has reported finding that in lean nondiabetic people, insulin tends to enter muscle cells, where it facilitates the use of glucose for energy. In the obese, however, insulin tends to go to fat cells and to make the fat person fatter. When an obese diabetic becomes lean, he may no longer be diabetic and insulin movement to muscles may be restored to normal.

At Pennsylvania Hospital in Philadelphia, when 800 men and women hospitalized for treatment of obesity were carefully tested, 57 percent were found to be diabetic or prediabetic. And many, when treated for obesity, not only lost weight but also then tested normal instead of diabetic.

Some physicians believe that a dividend from the discovery of the obesity-diabetes relationship is that it can help remove the stigma of gluttony and the guilt feelings many obese diabetics suffer.

Still another recent finding appears to have great significance. There has been a feeling that many diabetics, even if their disease is under good control, still run the risk of serious complications that must shorten their lives. But a recent study at the Joslin Clinic found 124 diabetic patients free of all complications after twenty-five years of diabetes. It appears that a significant factor in helping to prevent eventual development of complications is weight control. The mean weight of the long-lived, complication-free patients proved to be close to their ideal weights for their heights, and lower than that of the average man and woman.

What complications accompany diabetes?

It's an old story that diabetics may develop one or more of a considerable variety of complications, including eye disorders, skin and other infections, blood circulation disturbances, and pregnancy complications. More recently, such complications have been found to precede the appearance of overt diabetes in some cases. They may, it appears to some investigators, be the initial manifestations of diabetes.

That possibility first turned up in the pregnancy area. Why did some nondiabetic women have unexplained stillbirths, extremely large babies, and babies with congenital abnormalities, much as did some diabetic women? When the seemingly nondiabetic women were followed up long term, they were found to develop overt diabetes five, ten, and even twenty years later.

Then investigators began to note that some patients who developed cataracts, glaucoma, and other eye problems later became overt diabetics. And so did some others who experienced mysterious urinary tract infections, bladder disturbances, and inexplicable impotence.

The resulting new concept is that diabetes, instead of being simply a matter of high blood sugar, is really a general, complex, multifaceted disease process. Since such problems as pregnancy disturbances, eye troubles, skin and other infections—although long viewed as diabetes complications—did not necessarily depend upon the presence of high blood sugar over a prolonged period, they were concomitants rather than complications. Apparently, many changes could go on in the body before blood sugar became markedly elevated.

What is prediabetes?

The belief is that prediabetes is an extended state that may start early in life and continue until the day diabetes is discovered. During this period, structural changes may occur in the body that become apparent only after passage of time, a longer or shorter period of time varying with individuals.

Right now investigators are looking for tests sensitive enough to spot prediabetes. They are enthusiastic over the possibility that with early discovery of prediabetes and with treatment through diet regulation and possibly medication, the development of high blood sugar levels and other manifestations including obesity and coronary disease may be delayed or even prevented.

Can't prediabetes be detected right now?

To some extent, it may be. Physicians have been alerted to consider the possibility of hidden diabetes in a mother whenever there is an unexplained stillbirth, death of the baby shortly after birth, or an abnormal baby. And to consider the possibility, too, in cases of glaucoma, cataracts, kidney troubles of unexplained origin, circulatory disturbances, or other problems that might be associated with diabetes. When a relationship to diabetes is actually found, more effective treatment for such disturbances may be possible as the underlying diabetic state is brought under control.

How good are current tests for diabetes?

Quite good and getting better, and more is known about how best to use them.

The old test for sugar in the urine missed a considerable number, even as much as 80 to 90 percent of early diabetes cases. That's because during early diabetes the kidneys can still be working efficiently, taking sugar out of the urine and sending it back into the blood.

One commonly used screening test now is for sugar in a blood sample drawn two hours after eating. There are also more sensitive tests that can be used to confirm diabetes when it is suggested by the blood screening test and to check in doubtful cases when the blood test fails to indicate diabetes.

One such sensitive test is the glucose tolerance test, which calls for drinking a solution containing 100 grams of glucose (readily taken in lemonade, for example), then measuring blood and urine glucose levels at intervals afterward. Even more sensitive is the oral cortisone glucose tolerance test, in which cortisone is taken by mouth 8.5 hours before, and again 2 hours before proceeding with the glucose tolerance test.

Recently investigators have made another discovery about testing. Glucose tolerance studies have usually been done in the morning. But it now seems that performing the test in the afternoon instead may identify a substantial number of incipient diabetics who otherwise might be missed. At one center, 45 percent of patients who tested normal in the morning were found in the afternoon tests to have "afternoon diabetes." Some researchers believe that afternoon diabetes may be an early reversible phase in the development of carbohydrate intolerance and that, possibly, if people who have it avoid concentrated sweets, particularly at lunch, their afternoon diabetes may disappear.

Gout! That's a pain in a toe. What does it have to do with longevity?

Actually, gout doesn't have to involve a pain in a toe, although that's the classical site of attack. Gout can be a pain in any joint, or it may involve no pain at all.

Like diabetes and hypertension, gout is much more common than most people suppose; it's popularly misunderstood, and it's eminently treatable now. Common supposition holds gout to be the result of rich living, but that isn't true. It's often associated, on the one hand, with superior achievement. But it's also statistically associated with other disorders such as hypertension, coronary heart disease, diabetes, and obesity.

If you have gout, you may or may not know it. You can have it and think it's a kind of rheumatic pain. Or you can have elevated uric acid in the blood, which is associated with it—and have no symptoms at all.

Whether or not you have symptoms, elevated blood uric acid is associated with increased susceptibility to coronary heart disease, and that has much to do with longevity.

What exactly is gout?

It's an apparently inherited disorder in which there is abnormal handling of purines, which are compounds taken into the body as food and also produced within the body. Because of the abnormal metabolism, one product into which purines break down, uric acid, may build up in the blood and body tissues.

Uric acid is readily converted to a sodium salt, sodium urate. When that happens, the urate may lead to inflammatory reactions in a joint, producing swelling, stiffness, and pain. The joints commonly affected are those of the lower extremities, particularly the great toe, but any other joint in the body can be involved.

Sodium urate is also a major constituent of stones that sometimes form in the kidneys, and gout and kidney stones are closely associated. The incidence of kidney stones among the gouty is more than a thousand times as great as in the adult male population at large.

In advanced cases of gout, spurs or knobs of urate, called tophi, form and sometimes pierce the skin. There is a story of one man who could write on a blackboard with the tophi on his knuckles. Tophi themselves are painless, but they can interfere with movement of joints.

Is an attack of gout painful?

An acute attack is accompanied by agonizing pain. The affected joint—the big toe, for example—can look boiled, purplish red, so swollen that it appears to be inflated, with the skin tight and shining. It feels hot. But the agony lies in the deep throbbing pain, which is so intense that it's difficult to bear even the slight-est pressure on, or movement of, the joint. The English novelist Sidney Smith observed: "When I have gout, I feel as if I am walk-ing on my eyeballs."

How can gout be mistaken for anything else?

That big-toe attack seems distinctive enough. Even so, some people get such toe attacks and may think for a long time that they are somehow accidentally injuring the toe.

But acute attacks can strike in other joints; the instep, ankle, and knee are common sites. Two or more joints may be affected at the same time. Some people mistakenly think they suffer from rheumatism or arthritis.

Sometimes gout is present without any symptoms. Uric acid levels can be high; yet there may be no discomfort, no outward sign. In fact, some physicians report that by far the great ma-jority of cases are without symptoms.

Who gets gout?

Gout runs in families. Male victims outnumber females by about 20 to 1. The ancient physician, Hippocrates, explicitly asso-ciated sex and gout. He wrote: "Eunuchs do not take the gout, nor become bald. . . . A woman does not take the gout until her menses be stopped. . . . A young man does not take the gout until he indulges in coitus."

Knowledge of the incidence of gout even today is scanty. One estimate is that a million Americans are subject to gout attacks. The total incidence may be much higher.

For a long time gout was thought to be a rich man's disease because certain foods rich in purines—usually delicacies such as sweetbreads, liver, kidneys, and anchovies—are more likely than other foods to precipitate a gout attack. Their high purine content adds to the basic difficulty of the body in handling purines. It has long been known that a low-purine diet doesn't necessarily prevent attacks. Scientists have been able to demon-strate, using radioactively tagged foods, that people with gout tend to convert too large an amount of amino acids into uric acid.

Actually, somewhere in the course of evolution, man seems to have lost a particular enzyme that permits other animals to get rid of uric acid rapidly by changing it into materials that can be disposed of harmlessly. Even normal humans have a relatively high blood content of uric acid—about seventeen times as high, for example, as the dog. But people with gout produce still higher levels.

Is gout associated with superior achievement?

Alexander, Charlemagne, Galileo, Michelangelo, Luther, Calvin, Cromwell, Newton, Darwin, and Goethe are just a few of the distinguished men who were gout sufferers. But, of course, many other distinguished men didn't have gout.

Still, the association between gout and achievement has been persistently noted. In 1927, Dr. Havelock Ellis observed, "Genius is not a product of gout, but it may be that the gouty poison acts as a real stimulus to intellectual achievement."

More recently, uric acid has been found to be chemically related to caffeine and other compounds that can stimulate the cerebral cortex of the brain, which is more highly developed in man than in animals. The theory has been suggested that man's generally higher uric acid in comparison with other animals may have played a role in his intellectual development.

Some recent studies have shown that business executives have a markedly higher uric acid level in the blood than craftsmen. In one study at the University of Michigan, 113 professors were scored for drive, achievement, leadership, and similar qualities. Their uric acid levels also were checked. The conclusion was that the uric acid levels correlated closely with the desirable qualities.

How is gout linked with heart disease?

Cardiologists have recognized an unusually high incidence of heart attacks in gout sufferers. In a study at New York University School of Medicine, Dr. Menard Gertler found that among coronary patients "an astoundingly high number of them, 22 percent, showed high levels of uric acid in their blood."

How can gout be diagnosed?

It can and should be suspected whenever a man complains of pain and swelling in one or occasionally two joints which are sensitive to the slightest pressure. A simple blood test to measure uric acid level aids diagnosis.

Is treatment for gout effective?

Decidedly. Around A.D. 550 a Greek physician discovered that an extract of the meadow saffron gave prompt relief from an acute gout attack. Later, from this herb, a drug called colchicine was extracted. It is still widely used, and it is so specific for the treatment of gout that, when there is any doubt about whether a patient has gout, his response to colchicine can be a diagnostic clincher. If his symptoms disappear after a course of colchicine treatment, it is virtually certain that he has gout.

Colchicine usually stops an attack within twenty-four hours. Many people, able to predict the onset of an attack because of warmth and tingling in a joint, can abort the attack with colchicine. Moreover, colchicine has been used on a regular daily basis in small doses to prevent attacks.

Another class of drugs can promote the passage of uric acid through the kidneys. One is probenecid, first used late in World War II when penicillin was discovered but was in short supply. Probenecid was found to make a little penicillin go a long way. Later it proved capable of helping in gout. It sharply increases the disposal of uric acid in the urine so that the uric acid content of the blood may drop by as much as one-half. Probenecid now is often used in small daily doses, by itself and in combination with colchicine, to prevent gout attacks. Sulfinpyrazone is another useful agent that acts much like probenecid.

An even newer drug, allopurinol, actually blocks the working of an enzyme that converts compounds into uric acid. By reducing production of uric acid, it reduces blood levels of uric acid and thus prevents gout attacks. The drug also stimulates the breakdown and excretion of uric acid deposits that may already have accumulated in the body.

15

Checkups

Are medical checkups of any real value?

They can be. It is possible to discover many symptomless but urgent problems through checkups. Finding a few malignant cells on a Pap smear almost certainly can save a young woman from the ravages of cervical cancer. Early indications of a growing number of other cancers can be detected, including breast, prostate, and colon. In all cancer cases the earlier the discovery, the more likely the cure.

Early indications of diabetes and early signs and symptoms of emphysema can be detected, thus commuting the sentence of a man or woman otherwise likely to develop life-threatening diabetes complications or to cough life away. Treatment of a smoldering urinary tract infection in a person who didn't even know he had it can add years to his life.

Periodic health examinations range from a few simple tests for urine composition and blood sugar to elaborate complexes of tests aimed at checking on the functioning of virtually every body organ. So it's difficult to get any valid overall statistics as to the value of checkups. But some do come from carefully recorded programs of examinations for corporate executives. For example, the Mayo Clinic long has operated a checkup program for executives. Recently, a group of Mayo doctors reviewed the records of 569 executives from thirty-two companies examined over a twenty-five year period. In 474 executives, more than 83 percent, periodic examination had found evidence of disease. In almost 10 percent it was cancer; in 6.5 percent diabetes; in many cases it was obesity (and obesity is classified as a disease). Almost invariably, when the problem was something like cancer, the executive patients followed directions to the letter. When it came to obesity, only 15 percent complied well and another 24 percent complied partially. Still, the Mayo group concluded that periodic checkups produce definite benefits that make them worthwhile.

A more ambitious recent study, covering more than 20,000 examinations of male executives made in several clinics, arrived at the same conclusion. It found that the risk of death was reduced by nearly 50 percent in the regularly examined executives as compared with death rates in a comparable group of professional people not getting regular checkups.

Do all physicians approve of checkups?

No; some have mixed feelings. They argue that checkups may make some people morbidly anxious, and that their job is to heal the sick and not sicken the healthy.

The counterargument is that checkups for many people relieve anxiety; for others, they provoke thoughtfulness and efforts to improve health.

Addressing his brethren recently in a medical newspaper, one physician wrote: "The argument that we are more useful to mankind by attending the sick than by performing preventive medical examinations is emotionally soothing to many—but is it logical? If in older days all available doctors had attended the victims of smallpox epidemics, they would not have achieved even an insignificant fraction of the benefit of the activity of those who spent only a small part of their time with the vaccination of healthy people against this disease."

Many physicians who favor checkups note that it gives a good physician the chance to ask questions and give advice, a chance he wouldn't have if he waited for a patient to get sick; that if a checkup is skillfully handled, the patient should always go out feeling better. Says one physician: "First, the patient is encouraged to talk about a favorite subject, self. This seldom fails to make him feel better. Second, there is something wonderfully comforting about having your nagging doubts stilled by a doctor's verdict: You're healthy. The checkup also encourages the patient to get established with a specific doctor to whom he can turn in time of trouble. Likewise, it commits the physician to his care. It is the best way I know of insuring that when illness strikes, there will be a doctor on the other end of the telephone who knows something about you."

In spite of doctors who say they have their hands full taking care of the sick, there is increasing recognition of the need for preventive—and even prospective—medicine. It simply is not enough to do no more than treat the sick. That approach may have had some basis when the problem was infectious disease, and infection could be controlled with a wonder drug. But infectious disease kills far fewer people today and people live longer, allowing more time for chronic diseases to take hold. There are no easy cures for chronic, long-smoldering diseases.

What is prospective medicine?

Each person, when he is born and all through his life, faces certain health hazards. Many of these hazards that threaten him with early disability or death relate to his heredity, environment, personal history, age, sex, and color.

The physician can help the person meet these threats by making an individual health-hazard appraisal, based on regular checkups. The appraisal would take into account any slight changes shown by those checkups. It would also consider mass experience—what, on the basis of experience with many thousands of people, are risk factors for disease, and how important are they in general and in particular, given an individual's specific background.

The resulting individual hazard appraisal would be a determination of the individual's total risk situation and what has to be done to reduce the risks. That is "prospective medicine."

The appraisal would allow a physician to suggest that one person needs ten minutes more exercise a day or a change of job if possible and another needs twice-a-year checks for some specific disease he is much more likely to get than other people. In this way physicians could give their patients a better chance for survival, useful survival. It would be medicine practiced on the strength of probabilities of disease to come, of most effective means to prevent or at least retard the coming, and of means to minimize the consequences if and when it does come.

What is the basic idea of automated multiphasic health testing?

It's likely that prospective medicine is the medicine of the not-too-distant future. Its development may well be aided by the development of automatic multiphasic health testing. Such testing has immediate values for discovering disease in early stages; it takes a lot of the routine burden of testing off the shoulders of the physician; and if properly used, it can provide a lot of the mass data needed to determine disease risks and disease progression.

Automated multiphasic health testing aims to link detective devices, large numbers of chemical tests, and computer science to screen apparently healthy people at low cost. It provides physicians with the results of this screening and gives them more opportunity to counsel patients and practice preventive medicine.

One of the first steps in making possible such testing came with the development of automated laboratory equipment—robot chemists and other devices that could automatically carry out a dozen or more analyses on a sample of blood at the same time and could do multipart urine analyses. With this equipment it costs little more to do a full battery of tests than to do a single blood or urine test.

The results are sometimes startling. For example, automated laboratory equipment is often demonstrated at major medical meetings. Each year at the American Medical Association Convention an exhibit laboratory has been set up and physicians invited to have themselves tested. At a single convention as many as 2,400 physicians have served as subjects for such testing.

After five years of such testing it became clear that among men between the ages of thirty and sixty-five with living habits and occupation stress like those of physicians, about 20 percent will show abnormalities suggesting diabetes; about 30 percent will show cholesterol abnormalities deserving attention as indications of coronary disease; about 10 to 15 percent will show abnormalities that could lead to gout; and about 15 percent will show abnormalities pointing to kidney trouble.

What is automated multiphasic testing like now?

It's an assembly-line procedure. Generally, for a period of two to three hours, a patient moves from one station to another, where technicians, using batteries of electronic recording instruments, carry out tests for hearing, visual acuity, respiration rate, and lung capacity. A tonometric measurement is made for glaucoma, an electrocardiogram for possible heart trouble. A chest X-ray is taken and, for women, there may be a three-dimensional breast photograph (mammography). Pulse and blood pressure measurements are made; blood and urine samples are automatically checked for indications of infection, diabetes, gout, and other diseases, and also for various biochemical values that may give some indication of possible early or even predisease changes. The patient answers a self-administered questionnaire on health history.

Then a computer assembles, records, and prints out the test results in a form convenient for a physician to evaluate.

Do these tests really pay?

Judge for yourself. Aside from cancer and heart disease, at the Permanente Medical Group in Northern California, among 31,-843 men and women given multiphasic health examinations in one year, 17.35 percent were found to be obese, 7.55 percent to have high blood pressure, 7.3 percent to have anxiety states, 3.78 percent to have osteoarthritis, 3.33 percent to have diabetes, 3.33 percent to have gastrointestinal neurosis, 1.5 percent to have depression, 1.42 percent to have duodenal ulcer, and 1.34 percent to have migraine. That's a lot of ailing people among a seemingly healthy population.

Where is multiphasic testing available?

It's difficult to keep track. The U.S. Public Health Service has awarded funds to set up experimental programs in certain cities. Some of the programs are affiliated with health centers in poverty areas, others with universities, and still others, with city health departments.

Some large industries plan automated facilities as part of their occupational health programs. There are also plans for forming medically directed private companies to provide automated testing service for patients referred by physicians. As this is written, it is estimated that there are well over 100 centers now operating, and as many as 1,500 are expected to be in operation by 1980.

It is also estimated that about 10 percent of American physicians have become enthusiastic supporters of multiphasic testing; another 50 percent regard it as a useful tool; the remainder are opposed to it as a concept that may endanger the practice of traditional medicine.

In 1972 an American Medical Association report declared that automated multiphasic health testing "deserves thorough trial as a promising extension to the periodic health appraisals already conducted in general medical practice. . . . The procedures are not a substitute for physician services, but rather an exciting accessory to them."

Will there be improvements?

Unquestionably there will be improvements as more and better personnel are trained, as tests are increasingly refined, as new ones are added. For example, a new blood test allows detection of one of the most important forms of cancer—cancer of the colon—in its earliest stages, before it is visible by any other means. The technical basis for the test is such that there is some hope, and even conviction, among some researchers that the same test can be adapted for early detection of other types of cancer.

Multiphasic testing is still in its infancy. In any normal person there are scores upon scores of substances in the blood, others in the urine, still others in the saliva, and so on. The hope is to seek these out, determine the range of normal levels for them, and then correlate any departures from normal with subsequent development of specific diseases. Eventually, multiphasic testing may provide the very earliest possible indications of something about to go awry and what has to be done to remedy the situation.

As if to demonstrate that this is no impossibility, one new analyzer is capable, even at this early stage in its development, of separating out as many as 150 constituent substances from a single sample of urine.

How often should one have a checkup?

There are varying opinions. After an initial examination, repeat examinations at intervals of three years or more are adequate for an entirely healthy child and for robust people in their twenties. That advice is given by Dr. John G. Smillie of the Permanente Medical Group. He also advises that checkups are in order at two- or three-year intervals for healthy people in their thirties, at eighteen-month intervals for those in their forties, and yearly for people in their fifties and older. One important exception: women in the childbearing years and older should have limited examinations every year.

The American Medical Association leaves the question of frequency to the individual physician judging his individual patient, but suggests annual checkups for those over thirty-five, and also notes that a physician might want even more frequent checkups for people over fifty. The American Cancer Society favors annual checkups at all ages.

Certainly, it would be a good thing if even the minimum set by the Permanente physicians were met by most healthy people. But while there has been some increase in the percentage of Americans getting checkups, it leaves much to be desired. A recent nationwide sampling found that the percentage of those who *ever* went for a complete physical checkup when they were feeling well rose from 55 percent in 1961 to 57 percent in 1963 to 62 percent in 1970.

What should a checkup by one's own physician include?

There is no one set standard, and each physician may have his own idea of what should be included and how long a checkup should take. But, according to some authorities, a thorough scrutiny lasts at least an hour and anything less is only a rough screening.

There should be many questions by the physician, unless you are able to volunteer everything he needs to know. It can be helpful if you make a rough inventory in advance, including any important facts about your present and past health, any drugs you are taking or have taken, the kind of work you do, your travels, your family medical history, how well you eat and what, whether you are gaining or losing weight.

For a thorough checkup, you should be asked to disrobe completely. According to some authorities, not a single part of the body should be left untouched or unseen. Eyes, ears, nose, mouth, teeth, throat, skin, hands, feet, nails, armpits, joints, groin, pelvis, breasts, abdomen—all should be examined. Temperature, blood pressure, and pulse should be taken; there should be a chest X-ray and urine and blood tests, including a blood sugar test for diabetes (not just a urine test, which may miss early diabetes). And a rectal examination is vital. Too often it is skipped, though it can reveal cancer.

How can one find a good physician?

It's not easy for patients to judge a physician's skill, so the recommendations of friends or acquaintances don't necessarily mean much.

One way of proceeding is to phone a good hospital, or even several hospitals, in the community. Check with an administrator or a public information or public relations officer as to whether the hospital itself has a medical school affiliation, approval by the American Medical Association for training residents, or a certificate of accreditation from the Joint Commission on Accreditation of Hospitals. If it has any of these, it is usually a superior hospital. For example, Joint Commission accreditation means it is so organized that committees review the work of physicians and help to maintain top standards.

After you find such a hospital, ask for the names of several internists or family-practice physicians on the hospital's attending staff. An "attending" appointment indicates full acceptance of a physician by other physicians of the hospital, which is a helpful indication of good training and ability. Unquestionably, one of the best criteria for a good physician is that he have the respect of other physicians. If you happen to learn in the course of your search of a physician who serves as a family physician for many physicians and their families, he belongs at or near the top of your prospective list.

Once you have a list of several physicians, it makes sense to start with the one at the top and go see him. Have a physical. It's a good investment. If you decide to stick with this physician, it gives him a record of many things he needs to know if you should become sick and he has to treat you.

You may learn something valuable about yourself from the physical; you can learn something about the physician and your reactions to him: Do you like him? Do you feel a rapport between the two of you? Do you feel that you can trust him, confide in him?

You can observe him as he questions you in taking your medical history and then as he examines you: Does he take time? Is he thorough?

Your search may end right there. This may be your man. If not, repeat the process with the next physician on your list. It takes time and money, but deciding on a physician is a major decision.

After you've made your choice, you can continue to evaluate to help make certain your choice has been a good one. You can evaluate on the basis of how well organized his staff and office is. You can reasonably have second thoughts if you find that he seems content to just treat your symptoms without trying to find out causes or if he seems uninterested in preventive medicine through regular checkups.

What about having a medical checkup before undertaking any exercise program?

If you haven't participated in any extensive physical exercise since high school or college days, if your everyday work requires little or no vigorous physical activity on a regular basis—in short, if your life pattern is largely sedentary—you are "deconditioned." And before you undertake reconditioning, you need a check to make reasonably certain it is safe for you to do so and how best you can go about doing so.

Just what a physician should do—a set of criteria he can apply —in evaluating an otherwise apparently healthy individual for participation in an exercise program aimed at restoring at least a measure of the physical fitness of his (or her) younger years has been outlined in a 1972 report by the President's Council on Physical Fitness and Sports and the Committee on Exercise and Physical Fitness of the American Medical Association.

First, the physician must appraise the apparently healthy individual by a customary physical examination—medical history, known ailments, blood pressure, breathing, heart action, and so on. People beyond forty should get a somewhat more thorough examination than younger potential exercisers.

As part of the examination, the physician should test basic body actions both before and after a light exercise workout in the doctor's office. Once the physician determines that there are no conditions present that rule out exercise, he should then advise on a program of reconditioning that takes into account the age and present physical condition of the individual.

What kind of advice can he give about exercising?

A highly important aspect of beginning the exercise program, the report emphasizes, is to start slowly and gradually approach the desired level of activity. Exercise should be less than that which produces a degree of fatigue that will not be relieved by a few minutes' rest.

Initially, walking should be at a speed to cover one mile in twenty minutes. Later the distance can be extended to three miles to be covered in one hour. At that point, the pace can be increased so that the three miles will be covered in forty-five minutes. After that pace is achieved, most patients can progress to jogging.

The report stresses that the individual should set his own pace, even when he is exercising with others. Persons should be cautioned against feeling they have to keep up with a group. If unexpected symptoms occur, the activity should be stopped. If the symptoms do not subside promptly, there should be another physical examination by the physician before resuming exercise. The symptoms could be fatigue, anxiety, depression, chest pain or pressure, headache, dizziness.

The type of exercise is not the critical factor in reconditioning.

What is necessary is that the exercise produce an appropriate increase in pulse rate. Walking, bicycling, jogging, swimming are all good.

The activity should be enjoyable, otherwise it is likely to be abandoned. Routine exercise programs tend to pall after a few weeks. Group exercise programs, such as those of the YMCA and similar organizations, are more congenial for many people.

Finally, the report emphasizes, exercise programs are designed to improve health and achieve fitness and to assist in the prevention of heart and circulatory problems. For patients who have heart or circulatory disease, a program that has careful, continuing medical supervision is needed.

16

A Hard Look at the Major Killers

Is heart disease the number one killer?

Actually, the biggest killer is arteriosclerosis (hardening of the arteries), because it produces not only coronary heart disease and heart attacks but also strokes and serious kidney disease.

Diseases of the cardiovascular system—the heart and blood vessels—now take more than 1 million lives yearly, accounting for about 54 percent of all deaths. Cancer comes next, accounting for 16.8 percent of all deaths. Accidents take another 6.1 percent of lives. That leaves 23 percent for all other causes, everything from influenza and pneumonia to snakebite.

Some forms of heart disease, including congenital heart problems, have nothing to do with arteriosclerosis, and for these the outlook now is greatly improved. Such heart problems account for 16.2 percent of deaths due to all heart disease. Almost 84 percent of cardiovascular mortality stems from arteriosclerosis.

How has the picture brightened for other forms of heart disease?

Each year, some 40,000 children—blue babies and others—in the United States are born with heart defects. They may have holes in the wall separating the heart chambers, or they may lack proper blood vessel connections to the heart, or they may have valves within the heart that do not open or shut properly.

Only as recently as 1939 was the first successful surgical

operation for a congenital heart defect achieved. Now surgery can correct most of the major congenital heart defects. Even children with as many as four defects in combination are being helped. The chance for successful outcome of such operations ranges up to 99 percent. Moreover, for many milder congenital heart defects, nonsurgical measures now are often successful.

For rheumatic heart disease, too, the outlook has improved significantly. Rheumatic heart disease stems from rheumatic fever —and, even before the rheumatic fever, an untreated or inadequately treated strep throat. In about 3 percent of cases, particularly among young children, a strep throat is followed after several weeks by rheumatic fever that affects knees, wrists, or other joints. The most serious possibility with rheumatic fever is that it may inflame the heart and leave one or more heart valves damaged. Rarely is there serious damage after a first attack of rheumatic fever, but recurrences may cause trouble.

Fortunately, rheumatic fever can be prevented now by prompt use of a suitable antibiotic in case of strep throat. Moreover, if rheumatic fever does develop, recurrences can be avoided by routine preventive treatment with an antibiotic.

If, through neglect, recurrences lead to severe heart valve damage, surgical correction is often successful.

Syphilitic heart disease is preventable and curable with proper antibiotic treatment. Bacterial endocarditis, a heart-valve infection, once was 99 percent fatal. Now it has become 90 percent curable.

Acute pericarditis is an inflammation of the sac enclosing the heart; almost invariably, this disease can be overcome. And today, too, when myocarditis (inflammation of the heart muscle) occurs, it is rare that the patient cannot be saved, and the chances are great that he will recover normal function of the heart.

Is there any real hope for licking coronary heart disease?

Yes, there is. There's hope even when it is already present; treatment methods, including surgery, are becoming increasingly effective. Better yet, there is some real hope now for preventing it—for preventing the atherosclerosis that causes it and also causes strokes and serious kidney problems.

Is atherosclerosis different from arteriosclerosis?

Arteriosclerosis is a broad overall term meaning hardening of the arteries. The more accurately descriptive term used for the underlying causes of coronary heart disease, stroke, and kidney problems is *atherosclerosis*, which describes the thickening of the inner layer of the artery by soft fatty deposits called atheromas or atheromatous plaques. They look like pearly gray mounds of tissue on the inside of the vessel wall. Usually each mound has a core of fatty material, mainly cholesterol, covered by a cap of scar (fibrous) tissue.

Atherosclerosis is a slow disease. It may start in at a young age or even in childhood. The plaques grow slowly. There may be no symptoms at all for twenty, thirty, forty years or longer.

As the plaques grow in size, reducing blood flow in the affected arteries, tissues fed by these arteries suffer some deprivation. The coronary arteries feeding the heart muscle may be affected by atherosclerosis; in fact, of all arteries, they are most likely to be affected. But brain and kidney arteries also may be damaged.

What happens when brain arteries are affected?

When atherosclerosis damages a brain (cerebral) artery, there may be no symptoms if the brain area supplied by the artery is still receiving adequate blood supply via other brain arteries. Sometimes, even severe narrowing of a brain artery may cause no symptoms. But if the blood supply to the brain falls below a critical level, or if a clot becomes wedged in a narrowed artery and blocks flow, or if the artery ruptures, symptoms will usually develop.

The symptoms depend upon the area of the brain affected by the reduced blood supply. Various brain regions control various functions such as arm or leg movement or speech. In a stroke episode (sometime called apoplexy), there may be sudden loss of speech, or paralysis of a limb, or death. If started early, intensive medical care and protracted rehabilitation treatment can restore many stroke survivors to relatively active lives. Sometimes they may completely recover.

About one-third of patients who develop stroke do get some advance warning in the form of brief episodes (known as transient cerebral ischemic attacks) in which there may be one or more such symptoms as fleeting loss of speech, vision disturbance, loss of balance, dizziness, ringing in the ears, difficulty in swallowing, or weakness, numbness, or tingling of an arm or leg or the face.

If the symptoms are recognized promptly for what they are and are properly treated with suitable medication, a stroke may be prevented. A recent hopeful development is the finding that in some cases, the arteries that are affected lie in the neck region, where they are accessible to surgery, allowing restoration of adequate blood flow.

What happens when kidney arteries are affected?

If there is partial closure of one or both kidney arteries, the deprived kidneys may release increased amounts of a chemical called renin, which produces changes leading to high blood pressure. When the arteries become increasingly diseased, portions of the kidneys may waste away (atrophy), leading to reduced kidney function, which ultimately may have fatal consequences. It is now possible in some cases to surgically bypass blocked sections of kidney arteries.

Are there effects elsewhere in the body from atherosclerosis?

Unfortunately, yes. If atherosclerosis occurs at a point where the big abdominal aorta divides into two large iliac arteries to the legs, there may be cramps and pain in the thighs and buttocks upon walking. This condition is called intermittent claudication. If it becomes severe and incapacitating, surgery may be needed. If atherosclerosis occurs in arteries in the lower legs, there may be intermittent claudication symptoms, but usually the pain will be below the knee. Again, surgery may be needed.

When the disease affects the coronary arteries, are there always symptoms?

Not necessarily. The very first indication of the disease may be a heart attack, fatal or otherwise. In quite a few cases, the disease may lead to a silent heart attack, in which a small part of the heart muscle is deprived of blood and permanently damaged, yet the victim is unaware of it.

Thousands upon thousands of people, including young adults and even youths in their later teens, have atherosclerosis of the coronary arteries and don't know it; they have no symptoms whatever.

Isn't chest pain a symptom of heart disease?

Sharp pain, called angina pectoris, very often accompanies coronary heart disease, but not invariably. At some point in the progress of atherosclerosis, a first attack of angina may occur. Often, the victim is running for a bus at the time, or climbing stairs, or shoveling snow, or playing golf or tennis. The pain is constricting, like a steel vise tightening around the chest. It may radiate out from the chest to an arm (most often the left, but sometimes the right).

In effect, angina is a warning cry of the heart that it is not getting sufficient blood nourishment. For years the coronary arteries have been affected by atherosclerosis; slowly, as the disease has progressed, blood flow has diminished. Finally, the diminution reaches the point where some extra effort—running for a bus, for example—makes too much of a demand on the heart in view of its reduced nourishment. Angina is the signal. Usually it subsides promptly with rest or drug treatment.

Angina may be present for years in a stable state, getting no worse. Attacks may be brief and relatively tolerable. Medication such as nitroglycerin can quickly relieve an attack; and taken in advance of circumstances known to produce attacks, it may prevent them.

Sometimes, however, a patient with angina may die suddenly of a massive heart attack. Or the angina may become unstable, and the attacks occur more and more frequently, with less and less exertion or excitement required to bring them on. This worsening may indicate an oncoming heart attack.

What is the difference between angina and a heart attack?

In angina, the heart is temporarily starved. With a heart attack, a portion of the heart muscle, large or small is permanently damaged. The pain is similar to angina but usually much more severe, persisting for at least an hour and unrelieved by nitroglycerin.

What happens in heart attack is that a coronary vessel has closed off because of extreme narrowing or because a clot has formed and become lodged in a narrowed section, cutting off blood flow beyond that point. The site of blockage determines how severe or minor the heart attack is. If the closing off occurs at a point in the artery's course where blood supply to only a small part of the heart muscle is interrupted, the attack is minor. But if blockage occurs at a point where supply to a large area of heart muscle is cut off, the attack is massive. After an interruption of blood supply to a muscle area, the muscle at that site dies very quickly.

Are more heart attack victims being saved now?

Yes, when they can get to a hospital. About half of all deaths from heart attacks occur before the victims arrive at a hospital.

The deaths result largely from abnormalities of heart rhythm. Rhythmic heartbeat depends upon a smooth flow of tiny electrical currents across the heart muscle. They orginate in an area of the heart muscle called a pacemaker. The currents signal the heart chambers to contract. When an area of heart muscle becomes damaged, the current may no longer be able to get through it, leading to an abnormality of rhythm. In time, new current pathways are set up. But there may not be enough time if the interruption produces a severe rhythm abnormality that leads to heart stoppage.

Most hospitals now have special facilities in which heart attack patients can be monitored constantly with delicate electronic instrumentation. Instantly and automatically the instrumentation produces an alarm when a dangerous abnormal rhythm develops. In the overwhelming majority of cases now, prompt treatment— a quick shot of electricity may be used—can restore normal rhythm. Hospital personnel are always nearby to provide the treatment without delay.

The monitoring equipment is also capable of picking up abnormal rhythms that are not in themselves dangerous but are likely to lead to dangerous rhythms. These minor abnormalities can be quickly corrected with medication, minimizing the chance for danger to develop.

A heart attack victim who gets to a hospital still alive has an excellent chance of walking out again. Some efforts are now being made to equip ambulances with the same kind of instrumentation used in hospitals, with the hope of saving more lives. But there is no hope for saving the victim of a massive, instantly fatal, attack. And there is also the problem of educating people to call for help without delay when heart attack strikes.

Studies have shown delays on the average of from 3.5 hours to four or five days between appearance of symptoms of a heart attack and hospitalization. In some cases, the symptoms are not clear-cut. They may include what seems to be just indigestion, some dizziness, and shortness of breath. It's tragic but understandable that these victims may delay reporting their condition.

But, according to some studies, as many as 80 percent of heart attack victims who delayed for hours or even days had suffered intense chest pain and should have had some idea of what was going on. At one hospital, 60 percent of patients who were admitted with heart attacks had actually had warning signals, such as increasingly frequent and more severe episodes of chest pain for as long as a week before their actual heart attack, and had paid no attention to them.

The only good general rule is that anyone who has the slightest suspicion he or she is suffering a heart attack should get to a hospital as fast as he can.

Are there any ways of discovering atherosclerosis when it is not producing symptoms?

There are, but they are not simple. Newer diagnostic techniques, including electrocardiograms taken during and after exercise, increase the chances of detecting atherosclerosis before it produces symptoms. But the methods are still not as highly sensitive as they should be.

A special X-ray technique can detect atherosclerotic lesions. In this procedure a tiny tube or catheter is inserted into a blood vessel at a site such as the crease of the elbow and maneuvered carefully up into the heart, allowing a dye to be injected so the coronary arteries can be seen. The procedure of course requires hospitalization and therefore is not feasible as a routine diagnostic procedure.

Can surgery save people with advanced coronary disease?

Surgery looks highly promising. The first modern attempts to get more blood to the heart through surgery go back to 1945 when Dr. Arthur Vineberg of the Royal Victorian Hospital, Montreal, began to use the internal mammary artery as a supplementary heart-feeding vessel. The internal mammary lies inside the chest wall and can be spared, since other arteries feed the same area. Vineberg placed one end of the internal mammary in a little tunnel cut in the muscle wall of the heart. The hope was that the artery would hook up to unblocked branches of the coronary arteries. And after periods of six weeks to six months, this did happen in many patients, some of whom could increase their activities dramatically.

But some patients couldn't stay alive that long. Other surgeons devised techniques of opening blocked segments of coronary arteries and reaming out clogging material. Or they slit an artery and grafted on a patch of vein to enlarge the vessel. But both of these procedures were limited to the relatively few cases in which obstruction is confined to a short length of artery.

In 1967 Dr. René G. Favaloro of the Cleveland Clinic developed a new technique, using the saphenous vein, a large vein running the length of each leg. It returns blood to the heart but it can be spared because many other veins in the leg serve the same purpose. In fact, it is the saphenous vein that commonly is removed during varicose vein surgery.

Favaloro removed a section of saphenous vein, stitched one end to the body's big trunk-line artery, the aorta, and the other end into a coronary artery past the point of obstruction. Subsequently, other surgeons carried the procedure further, to the point where it has become possible to use two and even three short lengths of vein to bypass blocks in two or three coronary arteries.

This revascularization technique, as it is called, has the advantage of providing an immediate increase in blood supply to the heart muscle. It has been used in thousands of patients, including some with angina advanced to the incapacitating stage and some who already had had one or more heart attacks. The success rate has been above 90 percent. Risks accompany the operation, but the risks have been decreasing with experience.

The immediate results can be dramatic: patients previously unable to make a move without developing angina are now back at full-time work, free of angina, and able, after some training, to walk several miles and even jog. Hopefully, the improvement will be long term, but this remains to be seen.

Surgery, however, does not cure atherosclerosis. The atherosclerotic process, the burgeoning of fatty plaques in the arteries, is still there. Unless something is done to halt or retard it, it may cause serious trouble again at another site in a coronary artery, or in a brain or kidney artery.

What can be done after surgery to control the atherosclerosis?

The same things that can and should be done by heart patients who do not urgently need surgery and by those who do not yet have any overt atherosclerotic complications. Everyone should take a hard look at his risk factors, and then everything possible should be done to minimize the risk factors.

Do the same heart-disease risk factors apply to atherosclerosis affecting brain and kidney arteries?

They do. As blood cholesterol and triglyceride levels increase, atherosclerosis increases. High blood pressure, if untreated, adds significantly to the risk. The coronary arteries—for reasons unknown—are the most favored sites for atherosclerosis. But brain and kidney arteries are affected, too.

Atherosclerosis is more common among people with diabetes

or gout. There is increased risk of severe atherosclerosis among cigarette smokers. Behavior patterns and reactions to stress are also involved. Lack of physical activity is a major risk factor. Obese people have an increased risk of dying from complications of atherosclerosis.

Two or more risk factors are often present in the same person. People with three, four, or more make up an especially high-risk group. It is unlikely that all risk factors would be present in any one individual, but if they should be, he would have twenty-five or more times the likelihood of getting a heart attack, for example, than the average person.

Almost every one of the risk factors can be combated. Cholesterol and triglyceride levels, if elevated, can be reduced by diet, weight control, and exercise. If necessary, medications can bring them down. High blood pressure, gout, and diabetes can be controlled. Smoking can be stopped; short of that, a switch can be made from cigarettes to pipe or cigars.

Is it possible to have a near-normal life with a damaged heart?

After a heart attack, the body soon begins to make repairs. Part of the heart muscle has died; it can't be restored to life. But usually there is still plenty of good heart muscle left. The dead area of muscle is replaced by scar tissue, which after a period of four to six weeks becomes firm. Meanwhile, new electrical pathways have been established and new branch vessels, or collaterals, in the coronary artery system have been spurred to develop by the heart attack, so that blood is brought to areas around the damaged area.

After a time it usually becomes possible for the patient to begin to resume some activities slowly. An increasing number of physicians today encourage patients to avoid invalidism, to gradually resume many activities, to return after a time to work and to sexual activity. At some point, the physician may advise gentle exercise with a gradual increase in the amount. Exercise may help spur the development of still more collateral coronary vessels to increase blood supply to the heart. It can tone the heart muscle, enabling it to work more efficiently (see chapter 11).

Can further attacks be avoided?

Understandably, anyone who has suffered a heart attack has some anxiety that another will soon follow. But the risk of recurrence can be reduced materially. Exercise helps by making the heart more efficient, able to do more work with less effort. Weight reduction spares the heart. So does reduction of elevated blood pressure; and measures to reduce other risk factors are no less important and helpful. All of this holds true for recovered victims of stroke and the complications of kidney artery atherosclerosis.

The most effective way to deal with atherosclerosis is to prevent it. The most effective way to try to prevent it is to seek out and eliminate risk factors. This is the only way we have as of now, a way that seems logical and for which evidence of usefulness is beginning to accumulate. It is also the way that promises to be useful, even after atherosclerosis is well advanced, in preventing further advance.

What can be done about cancer?

Undoubtedly cancer is the most dreaded of diseases. An aura of fear and hopelessness has built up around malignancy. The common notion is that nothing can be done to prevent cancer; that once cancer strikes, the outlook is almost invariably grim; and that death from cancer must be agonizing. None of this is true, not that cancer is easily combated.

What's the current cure rate?

It could be 50 percent, but isn't. Yearly, in the United States, some 600,000 new cancers are diagnosed. About 200,000 persons are saved. Another 100,000 could be cured, but because of fear, apathy, and fatalism they are lost to the disease.

What's needed is a more aggressive attitude on the part of both the public and physicians. In this country 1.5 million people have had cancer and are alive today and, for all practical purposes, are cured. They have been alive for five years and more—in many cases, twenty or thirty years and even longer—after their bout with cancer, and they have had no recurrences and have no indications whatever of malignancy. Forgetting for the moment the fact that many cancers now can be prevented, the other vital fact is that they can be treated with constantly increasing likelihood of success.

Why, then, is there such pessimism about cancer treatment?

"The deaths in one's circle of acquaintances," one cancer specialist observes, "create their own melancholy publicity. The cures go unnoticed."

The most frequent reason given by cancer patients for failing to seek early medical care for symptoms that they suspect may be due to cancer is that the doctor, in fact, may find that cancer is what they have. They can't face up to the possibility of cancer because they erroneously believe that if they have cancer, they must die. As a result, far too many delay action until it is too late for new and effective cancer treatments to work.

The pessimism extends to many physicians, perhaps because during their training they are exposed largely to dying cancer patients in hospitals and have little if any experience during their training with long-term management of patients who respond to treatment and lead normal lives outside hospitals.

Perhaps the most important way is in the failure of some physicians actively to encourage their patients to get the regular checkups that would help to show up any cancer in early, most readily curable stages.

Only a few years ago, a survey of hundreds of physicians found that only 71 percent had ever *themselves* had an examination to uncover any disease that might be present though symptomless. Only one-third had had such an examination within the past year. As Dr. George T. Pack of New York, the cancer specialist who made the survey, observed: "It is hardly surprising that the public has not been spurred into action by efforts of health educators."

Have there been any really striking recent gains in curing cancer?

Many. For example, until just the last few years, Hodgkin's disease—cancer of the lymph glands—was considered virtually incurable. Now, in early cases treated with intensive radiation, a cure rate of 75 percent has been recorded, and even for more advanced cases aggressive treatment promises cure rates of as much as 50 percent.

Until recently, the five-year survival rate for the most common types of testicular cancer was 48 percent. Now 93 percent survival is being obtained. Cancer of the cervix, once a nearly unbeatable killer of women, is virtually 100 percent curable when detected in early stages, as it readily is with the simple Pap smear test. Breast cancer, the leading cause of cancer mortality among American women, claims 28,000 lives yearly. But at New York City's Memorial Hospital, records show that where the five-year survival rate for patients operated on prior to 1926 was 40.6 percent, it increased to 65.4 percent in patients operated on from

1949 to 1957. With newer detection methods—mammography (a special form of X-ray examination) and other procedures many more lives may be saved. In early, still localized, unspread breast cancer, there is an 85 percent survival rate.

Cancer of the colon and rectum, the most common internal cancer, takes 45,000 lives yearly in the United States. Yet it is known now that this type usually grows slowly, taking as long as 1,155 days to double in size. Of all such cancers, 90 percent can be detected in early stages, in time for complete cure, by routine annual examination. Even lung cancer, thought to be the most hopeless of all, curable at best in 5 percent of patients, is not that hopeless. Dr. Leo Rigler of the UCLA School of Medicine has reported that of 85 patients in whom X-ray examinations showed lung cancers 2 centimeters or less (1 inch equals 2.5 centimeters) in diameter, 53 percent are alive five years after surgery; in 178 others with cancers of 2.5 to 4 centimeters upon discovery, more than 40 percent have survived. "Such data," Rigler says, "contradict the extreme pessimism." Lung cancers only 2 centimeters in diameter are not, he emphasizes, difficult to detect. Even cancers less than 1 centimeter in diameter can be picked up.

Moreover, even when a cancer is not curable, when it has spread, it is becoming increasingly possible to use drug treatments to hold it in check. As one cancer specialist puts it: "Thirty years ago, the only true statement we could make to patients with disseminated cancer was, 'I can give you morphine for the pain, but no drug to work against malignancy.' Fifteen years ago, we could say, 'I can give you a drug that has produced some tumor shrinkage in some patients.' Today we can truthfully say, 'I will treat you with drugs and other agents, and there is a chance of long-term control of your disease.'"

What, basically, is cancer?

Cancer is wildly abnormal growth. The cells in body tissues normally behave in an orderly fashion. They reproduce to allow for growth in childhood and adolescence. They reproduce when new cells are needed to replace injured or worn out cells. If you nick your face in shaving or accidentally cut a finger, you can see how quickly the repair is made. Orderly growth of cells makes possible the healing of even large surgical incisions.

Cancerous cells, however, run wild. The normal controls over their reproduction are lost. Willy-nilly, without call for it, they reproduce repeatedly. If the wild growth is limited to one organ and does not invade other organs, the growth is called a benign tumor. Such a tumor may produce harm only through its size and the pressure it may exert on nearby nerves or organs.

Cancer, however, is malignant. It destroys the tissue in which it originates, eating into blood vessels, spreading to far-removed parts of the body through lymph or blood vessels.

What causes cancer?

There is still no definitive answer, but there are many theories. One holds that cancer is produced by viruses. The mechanism of cancer production by viruses might be this: In every cell there is a nucleus, which contains genetic material called DNA. DNA directs cell activities and also cell reproduction. Essentially, a virus is no more than a bundle of genetic material (often DNA) surrounded by an overcoat. To reproduce, a virus must enter a cell. When it does so, it drops its overcoat, and the genetic material invades the cell and then uses the cell's machinery to turn out more viruses. Cancer, conceivably could result when, under some circumstances, viruses invade human cells and upset the machinery in such a way as to make the cells reproduce themselves wildly.

It is also theorized that each person is born with latent viruses in his body cells—viruses that just sit there, causing no harm, but capable, when activated, of producing cancer. They may remain latent for a lifetime. But they may be activated when another virus enters the cell, or when there is injury from radiation or chemicals or other causes.

Does cancer always start in one organ?

Yes. It never originates as a generalized, bodywide disease. Some experts believe that a cancer may take as long as six years or more from inception to the point where it becomes large enough in a given organ or tissue to become obvious as a small lump. Its detection at the small-lump stage may still allow cure. If it could be detected much earlier, cure would be far more certain.

How can cancer be detected?

Cancer may be detected by actual feel, of course, in some cases. Various types of X-ray studies and biopsy—removal of a tiny bit of suspicious tissue for examination under the microscope—may reveal hidden cancers. Another method is the examination of shed cells, such as is done with the Pap smear test for cervical cancer and the sputum test for lung cancer.

There are warning signals—not certain indications of cancer at all but reasons for more intensive investigation. They include any sore that does not heal; bleeding from any part of the body when there is no obvious explanation for the bleeding; chronic hoarseness; chronic cough; unexplained stomach or intestinal symptoms such as constipation, diarrhea, nausea, vomiting, "indigestion"; unexplained pain; jaundice; impaired vision; and convulsions.

Any new detection tests that hold promise?

New tests may make many cancers detectable at much earlier stages. Among them are newer X-ray techniques, including mammography, which was mentioned earlier.

One of the most promising techniques—promising in itself and because it could open the door to a whole new means of early detection—is based upon a discovery made by Dr. Phil Gold of McGill University in Montreal. Gold established that cancers of the colon contain a protein substance called carcinoembryonic antigen (CEA). An antigen is any foreign matter in the body—a germ, a tumor cell—that stimulates the body to produce protective antibodies. CEA and antibodies developed in response to it have been found in the blood of patients with colon cancer.

Investigators in many laboratories are striving to develop a simplified test for CEA. They are progressing toward one that may be carried out in any hospital laboratory or even in a doctor's office. At the same time, other researchers find some evidence that a CEA test also may detect very early cancer of the prostate, the bladder, the lungs, the kidneys, and some malignancies of the nervous system.

Moreover, the discovery of one tumor-associated substance that can be detected suggests there may be other such substances. Some may even be highly specific for cancers at specific sites, allowing a cancer anywhere in the body to be pinpointed when it is still microscopic in size, very greatly increasing the likelihood of complete removal and cure.

Are there any practical ways to prevent cancer?

There are. They certainly cannot prevent all cancers or even most. But they can materially reduce the incidence of cancer.

The evidence is strong that elimination of cigarette smoking would prevent not only lung cancer but an appreciable additional number of cancers of lip, tongue, larynx, and possibly of stomach and urinary bladder.

Excessive exposure of the skin to sunlight is a known cause of skin cancer. This cause could be prevented by reducing exposure to sunlight and, if the exposure cannot be avoided, by covering the skin.

Radiation in excess can produce cancer. Special precautions are in order for people working with radiation. It's a good idea for everyone to keep a record of every exposure to diagnostic or therapeutic X-rays and to show it to doctor and dentist whenever new X-rays are suggested.

Some chemicals cause cancer. They include chromates, which may lead to lung cancer; aniline dyes, which may cause bladder cancer; asbestos, which may affect lungs or intestinal cavity. Anybody handling such chemicals or working around them should follow all safety rules.

In addition, certain premalignant lesions can be detected readily during regular checkups and can be removed before they have any chance to become cancerous. These include certain kinds of white patches on the tongue and lips called leukoplakia; senile changes in the vagina; skin conditions such as moles that begin to enlarge; and certain little outcroppings, or polyps, of the colon and rectum.

17

Is It Worth Living Longer?

Some people may cling to life—but is life worth living if it is vegetative or nearly so in the late years?

That depends upon individual viewpoint. But old age doesn't necessarily have to mean senility with its feebleness of mind and body. Much research today is directed at postponing or reducing the debilitating effects of age.

Isn't deterioration with age an inevitable matter?

Perhaps some of it is, but much of the deterioration once blamed on aging is really the result of disease.

One example is atherosclerosis, which was once considered a normal part of the aging process. But it is now clear that it has nothing to do with age per se. It's a disease. It can be found in young people, and it progresses with time. But time doesn't cause it. That understanding, replacing the older fatalistic idea of "What's the use, you have to get it as you get older?" allows a vigorous approach to establishing and then attacking the causes.

This is the modern scientific view of many of the so-called attributes of aging. Science has found that many of them come with age but not because of age.

What actual physical changes take place with aging?

From his twenties to his seventies, the average person loses about two inches in height. The body tends to become lighter because the bones lose some of their density and become lighter, and because body water tends to decrease. Some body cells may disappear and may be replaced by fat. There is wrinkling. There is also hair loss in both sexes: axillary hair tends to disappear; pubic hair becomes sparse; hair over the legs may disappear.

At birth the heart beats about 140 times a minute; it slows until age twenty-five when the rate levels off at about 70 beats a minute with the body at rest. But the heart rate is not the significant factor: how much the heart pumps, its output with each beat, is important. In a ninety-year-old that capacity may be only half as much as at age twenty.

Do all parts of the body age at the same rate?

No. Aging is something of a piecemeal business. A heart may fail while all else is fine. Kidneys may deteriorate and create disaster throughout an otherwise healthy body. Brain-artery hardening may produce mental senility in a still vigorous body.

Why do some people age much faster than others?

Some eighty-year-olds have been found to have a heart action —a pumping efficiency—as good as the average forty-year-old. Some individuals are senile even in their sixties or before and lead almost meaningless existences in their remaining years. On the other hand, there are many striking examples of creative accomplishments by the elderly.

People often point to Mozart composing his first symphony at age eight, Alexander the Great making his major conquests in his twenties, Keats writing his best-known poems in his early twenties, Albert Einstein publishing his first work on the theory of relativity when he was twenty-six. But consider, too, that Cervantes completed *Don Quixote* when he was nearing seventy; Goethe finished *Faust* at eighty-two; Verdi began *Otello* at seventy-two and composed his Requiem Mass at eighty-seven; Milton did not begin his greatest poems until he was fifty and blind; Sophocles was an octogenarian when he wrote *Oedipus Tyrannus*; Isocrates wrote his *Panathenaicus* when he was at least ninety-four; Titian and Michelangelo had long lives, productive throughout; Plato is said to have philosophized with his last breath; Beecham conducted orchestras without need for scores after he was well over eighty; Leopold Stokowski continued to conduct at eighty-nine; Artur Rubenstein at eighty-four continued brilliant piano performances; at ninety, P. G. Wodehouse published a new "Jeeves" novel, approximately his ninetieth book.

Are there examples of vigorous old age among
the less creatively gifted?

A *New York Times* account recently told of one man who sells lubricants to the petroleum industry outside Anchorage, Alaska; of another about to close "a honey of a deal" in negotiation for nearly eleven years from his base in Pennsylvania; a third who works eight hours a day but never gets so far from his Little Rock home that he can't get back before dark; and a fourth in Upper Sandusky, Ohio, who figures he is just getting started and has thirty more good years "before I call it quits." The first man is seventy-two years old; the second, eighty-three; the third, seventy-eight; the fourth, sixty-seven. They are among some 350 salesmen for a refinery company who are over sixty-five. This company, the Texas Refinery Corporation, makes a point of hiring older men.

Loma Linda University recently documented the fact that Mrs. Hulda Crooks, now seventy-five, still working as a full-time research assistant at the University's School of Health, had just completed her tenth annual week-long, 70-mile pack trip through the rugged High Sierra mountain range of California and her tenth 10.5-mile hike to the top of Mt. Whitney, the highest mountain in the continental United States.

Old age and illness don't have to go together?

Exactly. "We really don't understand the aged or the aging process, and so because there is a very high correlation between old age and illness, we have somehow got deluded into assuming that it's all right for old people to be sick," says Dr. Carl Eisdorfer, director of aging research at Duke University. As one example, Eisdorfer notes, "Some of our recent work on blood pressure and intelligence has pretty well demonstrated that what a lot of people have accepted as a normal process of aging—the loss of intelligence between sixty-five and seventy-five—is actually related to hypertension. In the group of subjects without hypertension, or where it has been controlled, we see no intellectual drop."

Dr. Don C. Charles of Iowa State University at Ames, after making a massive study of intelligence-test results, has concluded that performance in such tests improves from youth even into the fifties and sixties, with a little decline in some quantitative capacities thereafter balanced by continued verbal improvement; then age is no bar to learning.

Doesn't memory get worse with age?

Memory loss of some degree is frequent in old age. But it is *not* inevitable with old age.

Investigators at the Buffalo, New York, Veterans Administration Hospital have recently found that they can reverse transient memory loss in older patients by giving them periodic oxygen treatments. They have done so with seventy patients. Exactly what mechanisms underlie the success isn't known yet. Memory depends first on learning. It also depends upon storage retrieval, much like that of a computer. The greatest success of the oxygen treatment technique so far has been in patients with hardening of brain arteries. With oxygen treatments, the patients with such hardening appear to improve in storage retrieval. These results imply that much if not most of the loss of memory among older people is due not to aging but to artery disease, and that control of the disease could prevent memory loss.

Do older people lose their hearing?

They often do, but apparently such loss is not purely a matter of age. Dr. Samuel Rosen, a New York hearing specialist, has studied a Sudanese tribe, the Mabaan, and found that their hearing is as keen at age seventy as it is in most Americans at seventeen. There are indications that hearing loss in the elderly often may be related to artery hardening, possibly to the toll of long exposure to noise, and in some cases to thinning of the structures of ear bones essential for good hearing. Some investigators are now studying the effects of various substances, including fluoride, in preventing such thinning of the bone structure.

Is there any real optimism about prolonging the useful life-span?

Some investigators envision the future possibility of a human life-span of two hundred years or more. Many think the span can be extended to one hundred years well before the end of this century, and they are thinking in terms not just of longer life but of a longer period of active, vigorous life. Some approaches being investigated include the free-radical approach, cross-linking, autoimmunity, diet, the copying-error idea, and temperature regulation.

What is the free-radical approach to aging?

Free radicals are fragments of molecules. They can be produced by many things, including radiation, and they eagerly seek to recombine—in effect, to find new molecular homes. They may react with anything nearby. Free molecules, for example, cause butter to become rancid. To neutralize their effects and help preserve foods, substances called antioxidants are often used.

Free radicals are present in the body, and some investigators believe they may be involved in aging within body cells. Dr. Denham Harman of the University of Nebraska School of Medicine has found that free radicals play a role in the formation of amyloid, which is a fibrous protein that can be seen in increasing amounts in brain blood vessels with age, and also in areas of cell degeneration in brain tissue. Thus it is possible that free radicals may play a part in producing senility by damaging brain cells and vessels. By similar damage to other body cells and vessels free radicals may be involved in general aging.

This is still only a theory. Nevertheless, Dr. Harman has fed laboratory mice regularly on antioxidants such as vitamin E and BHT, the latter often used in breakfast foods as a preservative. In some mouse strains, such feeding has increased the average life-span as much as 50 percent. There is some hope that eventually the findings may be applicable to humans.

What is the cross-linking concept of aging?

Leather, rubber, human skin, and blood vessel walls have one thing in common: as they age, they lose elasticity. This loss appears to be the result of a process called cross-linking. In each case, the original elasticity comes from long fibers of a basic body-building material called collagen. With time, chemical cross-links form between the fibers, reducing their elasticity.

One theory holds that aging is a result of a gradual chemical cross-linking that goes on throughout the body in all cells. Actually, cross-linkages are always occurring to some extent. Most of the time, no harm is done since various enzymes, or chemical catalysts, in the body break the linkages apart as fast as they are formed. But a certain percentage of the cross-linkages occur in a way that prevents enzymes from splitting them. As more and more such linkages occur with time, normal cell functioning may deteriorate.

One investigator has likened the effect to what might happen if in a large factory with several thousand workers, two workers happened to become handcuffed together. The two, of course, would be able to do less work. If the handcuffing spread among other workers, even slowly, eventually the entire operation would come to a halt unless some way were found to uncuff them as fast as they became cuffed.

The hope is to find enzymes capable of breaking down those cross-linkages that are not broken down by natural body enzymes. One source for such enzymes might be soil bacteria. It seems likely to some investigators that soil bacteria contain suitable enzymes, otherwise the earth might well be covered with the undecomposed bodies of animals.

What is the autoimmunity idea?

The autoimmunity theory holds that the body's immunologic system, which protects it from disease, may undergo changes that make it cause aging.

The immunologic system provides antibodies that combat foreign invaders. Anything foreign—bacteria, viruses, even a transplanted organ—will stimulate the system to produce antibodies. Normally a youthful immunologic system produces antibodies that attack only foreign materials but not the body itself. But a number of diseases—including arthritis, myasthenia (a muscle disorder), and multiple sclerosis (a nervous system disorder)—may, it seems, be autoimmune diseases, so-called because they result from erroneous attack by the immunologic system on the body's own tissues. Aging, and perhaps still other diseases, conceivably may be results of such mistaken onslaught.

One study with mice used Imuran, a drug which suppresses the immunologic system and is sometimes used to give kidney and other organ transplants a chance to "take." When fed daily to mice beginning in late adulthood, Imuran extended the lifespan by about 10 percent.

Some investigators believe that the immunologic theory of aging may be compatible with the cross-linking theory. Antibodies, they suggest, may be cross-linking agents. If so, aging might be controlled by injections of enzymes from suitable soil bacteria to break down the cross-linkages as fast as they appear.

What is the diet approach?

In one study noted in an earlier chapter, hungry rats were found to be longer-lived rats. In a series of experiments, rats given unlimited calories were usually dead within 730 days. On the other hand, rats restricted to a diet of essential protein, minerals, and vitamins, with insufficient calories to maintain growth, remained in the preadolescent state for 1,000 days. When, thereafter, they received a normal diet that allowed them to grow, they matured sexually and lived longer. One rat lived 1,465 days, about the equivalent of 130 to 140 years in man.

More recently, Dr. Roy Walford of the UCLA School of Medicine has found that cutting the food intake of mice not only lengthened their life-spans but also made them less susceptible to cancer. Some of his low-calorie mice have lived to twice their normal life-spans and have shown significantly lower incidence of cancer than normally fed mice.

In other studies recently, investigators have used a synthetic diet—lacking in one protein building block, tryptophan—that stopped the maturing process for nine months in mice and chickens. When the chemical was restored, the animals started to grow again and lived twice as long as their normal life-span.

Certain other studies suggest an influence of diet on both aging and cancer, but it appears that the food intake must be limited enough to retard growth and must be kept limited throughout life, which would not make it attractive to humans.

What's the copying-error idea?

Every cell in the body has stored in its nucleus a set of blueprints for its operations. The information is coded into the DNA molecules that also govern heredity. Through intricate mechanisms the instructions tell tiny factories in the cell when and how to make enzymes, hormones, and other needed materials. Some scientists believe that over a long period of time errors may develop in the DNA system, leading to faulty material production, which is then mirrored by aging.

Such errors, or mutations, may be set off by chemicals and by radiation. It has been found that animals subjected to undue exposure to X-rays or radioactivity suddenly look older and get the usual killing diseases earlier.

Dr. Denham Harman fed mice a drug sometimes used for radiation sickness. They lived longer. Later, he fed mice compounds that appear to be somewhat similar chemically, compounds like BHT, the food-preservative antioxidant. These extended mouse life by 50 percent. So it may be that radiation and other influences set loose free radicals and the free radicals produce errors in the DNA system.

Some investigators believe that even when mutations in the DNA system are present, the cell may still harbor, in suppressed form, the blueprints that originally made it function properly; if so, a way might be found not only to eliminate the causes of mutation but also to reactivate the original valid instructions, and thus turn back the years.

How can body temperature regulation help retard aging?

There is evidence that body temperature has something—quite possibly a lot—to do with aging. Dr. Roy Walford at UCLA has found that he can double the life-span of some fish simply by lowering water temperature by 5° or 6° C.

At the National Institutes of Health, Dr. Charles H. Barrows, Jr., using tiny aquatic animals called rotifers, has established that when temperature is lowered from 35° to 25° C, the usual eighteen-day life-span almost doubles to thirty-four days. If, in addition, the rotifers are given only half the usual amount of food, they live for fifty-five days. Barrows has found that, at least in rotifers, there are two different effects: The reduced food intake extends the fertile, egg-producing period of youth while reduced temperature extends the later stage of life.

Dr. Bernard L. Strehler of the University of Southern California now has some cool eight-year-old mice of species that ordinarily have two- to three-year life-spans. A leading exponent of the low-body-temperature theory, Strehler feels it may quite possibly apply to man. He thinks there is some possibility that long-lived people may have slightly lower-than-average temperatures and that some study of whether they do or not is in order.

Strehler and others have investigated bats and other hibernating rodents and have found in experiments, that for every increase of 7° or 8° C in temperature, the rate of aging doubles; whereas with an equivalent reduction of temperature the life-span doubles.

If man reacts the same way, Strehler has recently reported, a reduction of 2° C could add fifteen to twenty-five years of useful, healthy life. Strehler believes that drugs can be found that may provide such reduction. Thus far, no ideal one is available. At the Institute of Experimental Gerontology in Basel, Switzerland, Dr. Fritz Verzar has tried novocaine, a local anesthetic. It does reduce animal body temperature, but it is unsatisfactory because it must be given in increasing dosages. Verzar urges further studies on other drugs that may safely cool body temperatures in mammals and possibly man.

Are there any other antiaging approaches?

Two others are getting some serious attention. One might be called the "shot of youth" approach. The other would hopefully increase life-span and retard old age by controlling body temperature.

The shot-of-youth method is based on injections later in life of certain cells taken from the body earlier in life. The idea is this: Scientists have long known that the efficiency of the body's immunologic system decreases with age. Fewer antibodies are produced; resistance to infection weakens. Only recently a team led by Dr. Takashi Makinodan of the University of Tennessee working with the support of the National Institutes of Health has been able to measure how drastically immunologic deficiency may decline. When they exposed mice to controlled doses of disease organisms, they found that old mice had one-tenth the capacity of young mice to fight off infection. In man, this may mean that a seventy-year-old is ten times as open to disease as a teen-ager.

The problem may lie, the investigators believe, with certain cells that produce antibodies. These are *T* cells formed in the thymus gland and *B* cells formed in the bone marrow before adolescence, which then become concentrated in the spleen and lymph nodes and also travel around the body as a tiny proportion of the white cells in the blood. When a foreign agent enters the body, a *T* cell and as many as eight *B* cells join to form an "immunocompetent unit" and in such combination produce antibodies. Recently, the investigators have found that the *T* and *B* cells, in old age, are not as efficient in recognizing foreign invaders. While the total number of *T* and *B* cells does not diminish with age, they may form only as little as 20 percent of the immunocompetent units, each turning out only half as many antibodies, as in youth.

But the investigators also have found that it may be possible to rejuvenate the old *T* and *B* cells. They have mixed old and young cells together and found that the old cells then become able to make antibodies at the same rate as the young cells do.

Already, in animal experiments, they have infected young mice with disease bacteria to stimulate their immunologic systems, extracted some of their *T* and *B* cells, frozen the cells for several months, then thawed them and injected them into old mice. Long after they had received the injections, the old mice were infected with doses of disease organisms lethal to other, unprotected old mice. They resisted the infection.

Possibly such a method can be applied to humans. First, however, researchers will have to determine if they can successfully freeze and restore live human *T* and *B* cells.

How far in the future are these techniques?

There is some rationale for all the work. Some of it may turn out to be totally impractical, some not. Undoubtedly, any relatively simple, feasible means of extending the useful life-span to 200 to 300 years, and even to 150 years, is some distance off. But it is quite possible that extensions of as much as 10 to 20 percent in useful life-span may not be so far distant.

The study of aging has suffered from a shortage of funds, which has been a severe limitation (in 1968 the federal government spent less than five cents per person to study aging). It has also suffered from lack of any practical way of testing possible life-lengthening procedures in humans. An experiment involving continuous use of even a harmless procedure that would have to last seventy or eighty years before there could be any evaluation of results is not very feasible.

But recently a whole battery of tests has been developed that promises to make it possible to carry out definitive experiments that would need to last only three to five years. There is some optimism among investigators in this field that trials with human volunteers will be under way within a few years.

According to Dr. Alex Comfort of England, a well-known investigator in the field of aging, "if the techniques used in rodents prove directly applicable, or if we have luck, then—allowing for the normal research tempo—some agent that demonstrably reduces the rate of mature human aging is likely to be known within fifteen years. The likely amount of such an increase, on the rodent analogy, could well be 10–20 percent."

Comfort goes on to note, "The limit of increase is not predictable at present because, for example, each increase gives additional time for research to bear fruit. The 10–20 percent estimate is based on the lower limit of speed in development, given present investment.

"If we should find that rodent-type procedures fail to affect human aging when started in adult life, or if the postponement of aging is partial, unequal, or accompanied by unforeseen effects, then the rate of progress will depend increasingly on the amount of research investment. However, once the machinery and experience for direct human experimentation has been created, new knowledge can be rapidly applied."

Are there any practical measures that can be used right now to help assure a healthier, firmer old age?

Yes, the same ones advocated for reducing the risks of such killer diseases as coronary heart disease and strokes. They also have applicability for avoiding many failings once mistakenly thought to be inevitable with aging.

Controlling high blood pressure, for example, at once controls a major factor in atherosclerosis and, as recent research has shown, a major factor in intellectual decline after sixty-five. And if memory deficit is linked with oxygen shortage in the brain, as recent research suggests, the measures to control atherosclerosis, which is linked with reduced blood and oxygen flow, may well minimize or avoid memory impairments.

Exercise is another measure that, in addition to helping retard or prevent atherosclerosis, may help ward off some of the characteristics of many older people that have nothing to do with aging. Says Dr. Fred Schwartz, chairman of the American Medical Association Committee on Aging: "Many so-called infirmities of age stem directly from lack of conditioning. Great numbers of individuals, after leaving high school or college, settle down to a routine of breadwinning that uses only a small portion of their muscle or physical equipment. In these circumstances, it is easy to understand why physical horizons have become cramped and why hands shake and why the gait becomes uncertain and tottery."

Wrinkling comes with age, but a recent study has found that it comes more quickly with smoking. The study, covering 1,104 subjects, found a striking association, in both men and women, between the degree of wrinkling and the duration and intensity of smoking. Smokers, beginning even as early as age thirty, are as likely to be as prominently wrinkled as nonsmokers twenty years older.

Dr. Nathan W. Shock, chief of the Gerontology Research Center of the Department of Health, Education, and Welfare, has recently reported that the lung function of chronic cigarette smokers is, on the average, reduced to levels of nonsmokers who are approximately ten years older. But when an individual stops smoking, in twelve to eighteen months his lung function may return nearly to the levels of nonsmokers; this applies even to sixty-year-olds. Recuperative processes are still active in older people.

Even researchers convinced that a massive cutback in food consumption could do much to extend life don't see near-starvation as a practical approach. But they argue that most of us need to cut back on our overeating as a matter of girth control and moderation of eating could be a favorable factor for vigorous later years.

Insults to the body may accelerate aging. They include the undue stress from long-continued tension and anxiety and from long-continued chronic infection or other conditions amenable to treatment. "Every stress," says Dr. Hans Selye of the Institute for Experimental Medicine and Surgery at the University of Montreal, "leaves an indelible scar, and the organism pays for its survival after a stressful situation by becoming a little older." If this is the case, prompt attention to any illness, refusal to delay treatment, may do more than save needless discomfort. So may learning to relieve anxiety and tension through physical activity and other measures discussed earlier.

Will we ever be satisfied with the length of the human life-span?

Perhaps. Perhaps not. Elie Metchnikoff, a great biologist whose fundamental studies on infection and immunity won him the Nobel Prize, turned his attention later in life to old age.

As René Dubos has pointed out, Metchnikoff "wondered why men fear death and often show anxiety at its approach. Every function [Metchnikoff observed] calls into play an instinct of satiety; a satisfying meal leaves us without desire for further food; we look forward to rest after sufficient exertion. Why, then, do we not experience a desire for death at the end of a normal life?

"It is, Metchnikoff thought, because human life is usually much shorter than the number of years of which it is potentially capable. Human beings who reach a really ripe age—say 100 years or more—do welcome death without regrets even though they are not sick and do not suffer, just as the normal person welcomes sleep at the end of a full day."

18

Your Personal
Inventory

So here you are, a person not quite like any other. How long your life will last and how healthy and vigorous it will be is being influenced by many factors that, in their specific combination for you, form a distinctive pattern.

The chart that follows is intended to help you draw up a personal inventory, a graphic representation of the factors operating in your life. Hopefully it will give you a better total picture of your strengths and weaknesses, and warn you of any factors that may be increasing your risk of heart attack, stroke, cancer, or other disease. It can serve as a guide to reducing the risk of such disease and, by so doing, increase the likelihood of a longer and continuously more vigorous and healthy life.

How to prepare the inventory

The various influences, with references to the chapters in which they are discussed, are listed on the chart. If you have not already done so in your first reading, you can refer back to the individual chapters to pick out information applying to yourself and then make use of it on the chart.

For example, is your family history one of remarkable health? Is yours an extremely long-lived set of progenitors, free of disease and vigorous until very late in life? If so, you would certainly

PERSONAL INVENTORY

CHAPTER REFERENCE	INFLUENCE	INCREASED RISK FOR HEART ATTACK STROKE CANCER OTHER			
2	Family history				
3	Sex				
4	Childhood and early influences				
5	Body type				
5	Intelligence				
5	Education				
6	Where you live				
7	Work				
7	Income				
7	Marital status				
8	Personality				
9	Sex life				
10	Weight				
11	Physical activity				
12	Diet				
13	Smoking				
13	Drinking				
13	Sleeping				
13	Relaxation				
14	Blood pressure				
14	Diabetes				
14	Gout				
15	Medical checkups				

have no increased risk—on the basis of family history—for early serious disease and shortened life.

On the other hand, if certain diseases have been prominent in the family, you may run some increase in risk of developing them, on a genetic or family predisposition basis. If so, you should check the appropriate box (heart attack, stroke, cancer) or write under "other" what the disease is.

Neither sex is immune to serious disease and premature death. Women seem to have an innate advantage for living longer, everything else being equal. But while men are more prone to some diseases, there are others to which women are more prone. On the basis of your sex, you can indicate increased risks for specific diseases.

Similarly, you can take into account childhood and early influences (including season and order of birth), body type, intelligence, education, place of residence, type of work, income, and marital status. As you will have noted in the chapters covering these subjects, each may have some bearing on risk and you can note on the chart which, if any, may in your case make for increased risk and for which disease.

As you will also have noted in the respective chapters, the other influences listed on the chart—from personality through medical checkups—may increase risk for sickness and shortening of life. How, from your examination of the known facts about these influences and from your knowledge of yourself, do you rate? Which of these are operating in your life to increase your risk for disease? You can make appropriate notations on the chart.

Your priorities

Once you have filled in the chart, you should be able to see clearly the risk-increasing influences in your life. And you may well have a good idea what your priorities should be to reduce risks and increase the likelihood of living a longer, healthier life.

Increased risk need not predict an inevitable outcome. For example, if your family has a history of early deaths from heart disease, you may be somewhat more likely than another person to have trouble with heart disease, everything else being equal. But everything else need not be equal. While family predisposition is not to be dismissed lightly, it is far from being an overriding influence. If all or most other influences are, or can be made, favorable, family predisposition may be completely eclipsed.

Most encouraging, too, is the fact that risk factors often interact. They affect each other. Controlling one often helps to bring one or more others under control. If, for example, you are at risk because of high blood pressure, obesity, and lack of exercise, you may need only a suitable exercise program to solve the obesity problem and, in the process of solving the obesity problem, you may also solve the problem of elevated blood pressure.

You cannot, of course, change such influences as heredity, sex, and order or season of birth. But there are the many influences that, if harmful, can be changed. In a sense, you can look upon the problem as being somewhat like wanting to keep a boiling, full pot from overflowing. You can moderate the flame or spoon off some of the contents; you don't necessarily have to change the pot or start all over again with new ingredients.

After filling out the chart your first step should be to get a thorough medical checkup unless you have had one in recent months. For one thing, you should know the present status of your blood pressure and blood fats, whether you have gout or diabetes in a nonobvious form, and the condition of your heart and other vital organs. If treatment is needed for any of these, you should have it now. Delay only adds insult to the body.

Your physician, moreover, should be able to help you with specific advice on desirable changes in your way of life. He can reinforce your confidence by approving, based on his latest findings of your condition, any program you draw up for yourself based on guidelines and suggestions offered in the earlier chapters of this book. If necessary, he may counsel on modifying your program to make it more suitable for you. You have a right to expect such guidance and help.

There is going to be a change in medicine—in the role of the physician. "Looking honestly at the present," Dr. William H. Steward, former surgeon general of the U.S. Public Health Service, observed recently, "we have to acknowledge that preventive medicine is in a state of partial eclipse. . . . Especially in the two decades since World War II, medicine has been in a therapeutic era. The accent has been on diagnosis, treatment, and cure. The glamor fields have been those associated with cure and repair, like surgery and chemotherapy. None of us would deny the brilliant accomplishments . . . at a price. The thrust . . . has required specialization [which] has led to compartmentalized knowledge . . . and practice. Our concern with the human being has been fragmented. And he, after all, is the purpose of the whole endeavor. . . . The individual has been placed outside the system. . . . It sometimes seems that he is being asked to shed his community, his family, and his 'self' in the process, so that the physician can get down to the piece of action he is mainly interested in. In my view, the revolutionary change needed in our health system is to reorient it to the human being. The individual, as a person, should be the center around which the service system revolves, his total state of health its measure of success or failure."

Not long ago Dr. Gerald Besson, president of a California medical society, made these keen observations: "The environment's hazards are physical, biological, or sociocultural. Our defenses are genetic, learned, or involve external assistance. The bulk of the interaction between self and environment takes place without medical care intervention. Indeed, it is only a minute segment of this endless encounter that involves medical care. Much of the interaction may be influenced in favor of the host by certain acts by either the individual—if he knows how—or by a professional.

"In the framework of this definition the profession changes its emphasis. We deal more with people and less with patients. We deal more with health than with disease. We deal more with the human condition, less with formalin-fixed pathology. We deal more with sociocultural hazards than with the biological ones. We deal more with a continuum of care, less with the episode of sickness."

Medicine, of course, must continue to fight disease when it appears. But it must become—and already is starting to become—more concerned with preventing its appearance, with caring for the well to maintain health.

Health takes more than doctors and dollars. Health is too important to be left to doctors, even if it could be. Health, ultimately, is an individual matter, a very personal thing. It requires, first of all, the attention and concern of the individual. Only then can doctors be of real help.

The most important factor in health and longevity is for the individual to understand what he needs to do in his own interest and then to do it.

Further Reading

Berland, Theodore. *The Fight for Quiet*. Englewood Cliffs, N.J.: Prentice-Hall, 1970.
————. *Biological Rhythms in Psychiatry and Medicine*. Bethesda, Md.: National Institute of Mental Health, 1970.
Calder, Nigel. *The Mind of Man: An Investigation into Current Research on the Brain and Human Nature*. New York: Viking Press, 1971.
Claiborne, Robert. *Climate, Man and History*. New York: Norton, 1970.
Cohen, Martin. "How the Heavens Influence Our Lives." *Today's Health*, October 1971.
Crew, F. A. E. *Health: Its Nature and Conservation*. Oxford and New York: Pergamon Press, 1965.
Critchfield, Howard J. *General Climatology*. Englewood Cliffs, N.J.: Prentice-Hall, 1966.
Darlington, Cyril Dean. *The Evolution of Genetic Systems*. New York: Basic Books, 1958.
Dobzhansky, Theodosius G. *Heredity and the Nature of Man*. New York: Harcourt, Brace & World, 1964.
Dubos, René. *Mirage of Health*. New York: Harper & Row, 1959.
————. *So Human an Animal*. New York: Charles Scribner's Sons, 1968.
Emery, Alan E. *Heredity, Disease and Man: Genetics in Medicine*. Berkeley: University of California Press, 1968.
Forrester, Frank H. *1001 Questions Answered About the Weather*. New York: Dodd, Mead, 1957.
Fox, John P.; Hall, C. E.; and Elveback, L. R. *Epidemiology: Man and Disease*. New York: Macmillan, 1970.
Fox, Robin. "Chinese Have Bigger Brains Than Whites—Are They Superior." *The New York Times* magazine, June 30, 1968, p. 13.
Gallup, George, and Hill, Evan. *The Secrets of Long Life*. New York: Bernard Geis Associates, 1960.
Galton, Lawrence. *The Silent Disease: Hypertension*. New York: Crown Publishers, 1973.
Galton, Lawrence. *Don't Give Up on an Aging Parent*. New York: Crown Publishers, 1975.
Glemser, Bernard. *Man Against Cancer*. New York: Funk & Wagnalls, 1969.
Handler, Philip, ed. *Biology and the Future of Man*. New York: Oxford University Press, 1970.
Harrington, Alan. *The Immortalist*. New York: Random House, 1969.
Hunt, Morton M. *The Thinking Animal*. Boston: Little Brown, 1964.
Klein, Aaron E. *Threads of Life: Genetics from Aristotle to DNA*. New York: The Natural History Press, 1970.
Knudson, Alfred G. *Genetics and Disease*. New York: McGraw-Hill, 1965.
Landsberg, H. E. *Weather and Health: An Introduction to Biometeorology*. Garden City, N.Y.: Doubleday, 1969.

Lewis, H. R., and Lewis, M. E. *Psychosomatics: How Your Emotions Can Damage Your Health.* New York: Viking Press, 1972.

Likoff, W.; Segal, B.; and Galton, L. *Your Heart: Complete Information for the Family.* Philadelphia, Pa.: J. B. Lippincott, 1972.

Lowry, William P. *Weather and Life.* New York: Academic Press, 1969.

Miller, B. F., and Galton, L. *Freedom from Heart Attacks.* New York: Simon & Schuster, 1972.

———. *The Family Book of Preventive Medicine.* New York: Simon & Schuster, 1971.

McGrady, Patrick M., Jr. *The Youth Doctors.* New York: Coward-McCann, 1968.

McKusick, Victor A. *Mendelian Inheritance in Man.* 3rd ed. Baltimore: Johns Hopkins Press, 1971.

McQuade, Walter. "What Stress Can Do to You." *Fortune,* January 1972, p. 102.

Mather, William G., and others. *Man, His Job, and the Environment: A Review and Annotated Bibliography of Selected Recent Research on Human Performance.* Washington, D.C.: National Bureau of Standards Special Publication 319, U.S. Government Printing Office, 1970.

Mayer, Jean. *Overweight: Causes, Cost, and Control.* Englewood Cliffs, N.J.: Prentice-Hall, 1968.

Neff, W. S. *Work and Human Behavior.* New York: Atherton Press, 1968.

Newman, E. V., and others. *Arteriosclerosis: A Report by the National Heart and Lung Institute Task Force on Arteriosclerosis.* Vols. 1 and 2. DHEW pub. no. (NIH) 72-137. Washington, D.C.: U.S. Government Printing Office, 1972.

Porter, Ian H. *Heredity and Disease.* New York: McGraw-Hill, 1968.

Prehoda, Robert W. *Extended Youth.* New York: G. P. Putnam's Sons, 1968.

Rose, C. L., and Bell, B. *Predicting Longevity: Methodology and Critique.* Lexington, Mass.: Heath Lexington Books, 1971.

Scheinfeld, Amram. *Heredity in Humans.* Philadelphia: J. B. Lippincott, 1971.

———. *Your Heredity and Environment.* Philadelphia: J. B. Lippincott, 1965.

Sheldon, W. H. *Atlas of Men: A Guide for Somatotyping the Adult Male at All Ages.* New York: Harper & Row, 1954.

———. *The Varieties of Human Physique: An Introduction to Constitutional Psychology.* Darien, Conn.: Hafner Pub. Co., 1970.

Smith, Anthony. *The Seasons.* New York: Harcourt, Brace, Jovanovich, 1970.

Smoking, The Health Consequences of: A Report to the Surgeon General. Washington, D.C.: U.S. Department of Health, Education and Welfare, 1971.

Winchester, Albert McC. *Genetics: A Survey of the Principles of Heredity.* 3rd ed. Boston: Houghton Mifflin, 1966.

Index

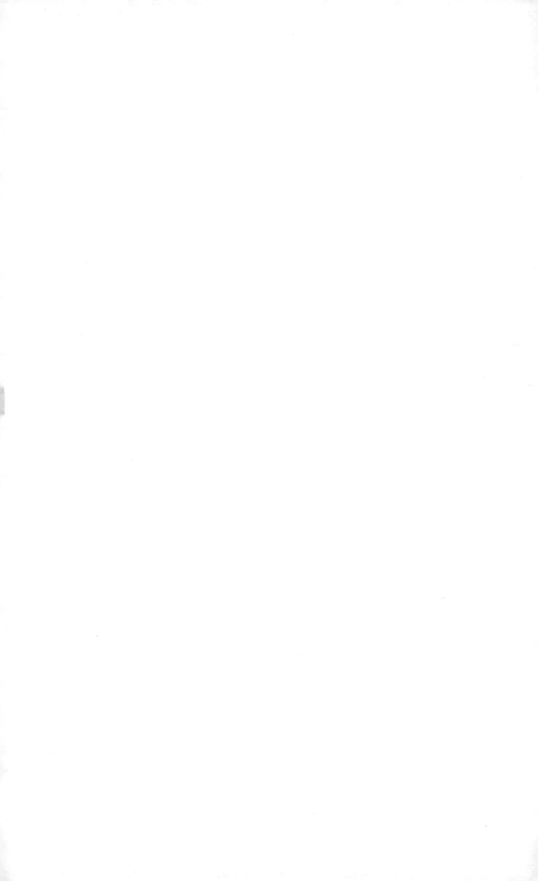

Index

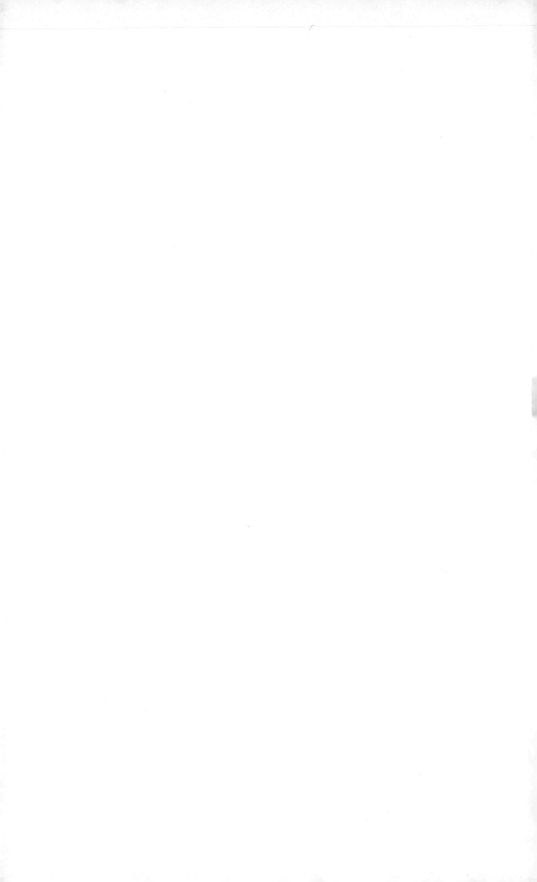